Robert H. Kelsoe

Recommended by Don Peterson 2006

The Nun and the Bureaucrat

HOW THEY FOUND AN UNLIKELY CURE FOR AMERICA'S SICK HOSPITALS

Louis M. Savary
and Clare Crawford-Mason

CC-M Productions, Inc.
2006

For information about permission to reproduce selections
from this book, contact:

CC-M Productions, Inc.
7755 Sixteenth Street, N.W.
Washington, D.C. 20012
(202) 882-7430
www.ManagementWisdom.com

Book design & layout by Victor Crawford, Jr.

Library of Congress Cataloguing-in-Publication Data

Savary, Louis M.
The Nun and the Bureaucrat:
How They Found an Unlikely Cure for America's Sick Hospitals/
Louis M. Savary and Clare Crawford-Mason.

ISBN 0-9779461-0-X

1. Hospitals. 2. Health Care. 3. Total quality management.
I. Crawford-Mason, Clare. II. Title.

Printed in the United States of America

DEDICATION

This book is dedicated to Herbert E. Striner, former dean of the Kogod School of Business, The American University. He began the introduction of these vital ideas to the Western world when he sent the producers of "**If Japan Can...Why Can't We?**" to see W. Edwards Deming in 1979;

And to Jefferson Vander Wolk, hotel and restaurant operator, who has successfully pioneered the use of systems thinking by employees to keep upgrading their personal success skills on the job and off.

Contents

FOREWORD

"Once upon a time," may be the four most powerful words in the English language. They capture attention and introduce a story, which is the best way to explain a new and complicated idea, especially an idea that refutes conventional wisdom

This book reports such a story—told by doctors, nurses and hospital administrators—of how a new idea, called "systems thinking," helped to transform the way they understood and organized their work and allowed them to dramatically improve over sixty sick hospitals: saving lives and reducing costs and patient suffering.

Astounding and significant as that is, the story also offers a solution to America's biggest and most pressing domestic problem: healthcare. Every lawmaker, civic leader, employer and informed citizen knows four facts about healthcare: (1) healthcare is the biggest domestic problem they face; (2) healthcare financing costs are spiraling out of control; (3) many millions of Americans have no health insurance; and (4) these leaders do not agree or know how to fix these problems.

More and more Americans are aware of another four facts: (1) that personal and family healthcare costs are crippling; (2) that as hospital patients they are not the center of attention; (3) that hospitals are dangerous places because hospital-acquired infections are among the top five causes of death in the United States; and (4) that people feel helpless about this and have no idea what to do to improve the situation. Many hospital administrators, physicians, and nurses know four additional facts: (1) that most American hospitals are sick; (2) that they are crippled by inadequate and outdated management practices, unnecessary duplication of services and astounding waste; (3) that hospitals generate many avoidable, often deadly, mistakes—including countless "near misses," that is, mistakes that almost happened; and (4) that it is in hospitals where the turnaround in healthcare costs and safety must begin.

Like any great change, it begins with a new idea, one which we said, defies conventional wisdom.

The compelling and urgent impetus behind our book and its com-

I

panion PBS documentary is more than significantly increased patient safety and reduced healthcare costs, as important as they are. It is the story of an important new idea, systems thinking. It is a story of how systems thinking could be transported from the factory floor of an automobile plant and used to improve safety and costs. We believe it is crucially important for all Americans to understand systems thinking, realize its immediate practicality, and recognize that it is being successfully used in improving organizations from schools to hospitals to government offices, manufacturing plants and families. Many more urgently need it.

Here is a summary of the story.

> Once upon a time, there were two hospital systems, one run by a nun, the other led by a bureaucrat. Their doctors, nurses and administrators were well educated and deeply committed to healing the sick. They did their best and worked overtime trying to improve the healthcare services they provided. Yet things kept getting worse.
>
> Every day, more and more patients acquired new infections at the hospitals. There were medical errors. Patients suffered and died unnecessarily. Enormous wastes of time and supplies and potential errors were hidden in traditions, habits and conflicting regulations. Costs kept spiraling upward, mistakes kept happening, and the healthcare professionals and administrators were ever more concerned and frustrated.
>
> They knew they were not alone because they saw a steady stream of books, magazines and newspapers reporting that U.S. hospitals are expensive and dangerous, potentially deadly places.
>
> Their situation seemed hopeless. However, the leaders were open to new ideas.
>
> Administrators at one Midwest hospital system in the late 1980s found out about systems thinking and began to use it. It worked. Deaths, suffering, waste and errors were reduced. In the late 1990s a group of hospitals in Pittsburgh joined with insurance companies and employers to try to improve their services, while they still competed for patients.

II

How they did it is one of the most fascinating parts of the story. They found an auto manufacturer who taught them systems thinking and its new way of looking at their work. Patient safety began to improve dramatically. Doctors and nurses in both hospital systems reported they found their work more rewarding.

SYSTEMS THINKING

The term "systems thinking" may sound complicated and technical, as if only scientists or mathematicians could grasp it. However, you don't need a college degree to understand systems thinking.

When applied to a complex organization such as a hospital, systems thinking simply means focusing on the organization as a whole—and transforming it as a whole—rather than paying attention only to its various parts or departments. This is what the doctors, nurses, and administrators in our story learned to do. Instead of just concentrating on their own job, typical of people in most organizations, they began looking at how all of the different people and technological devices in their hospitals worked together on behalf of the patient. Once these people learned systems thinking, they applied it to heal sickness, reduce failure and mistakes, and eliminate waste at every level in their hospitals.

In this book, doctors, nurses, administrators, aides—regular people—tell in their own words how they overcame doubts that they could provide "perfect patient care," identify errors, reorganize how they worked together, learn a new systems way of thinking, develop "new eyes" to design better and better methods, and get to the roots of problems.

Systems thinking is not a panacea that can erase every mistake, but it is a tool for seeing a world that can be improved and solving many organizational problems. In this way, it helps create a society better able—than it has been—to deal with the constant changes and growing complexity in our 21st Century world.

UNCERTAIN WORLD

One hundred years ago, most people accepted that the world was an uncertain place in which extreme weather, disease, and political events unexpectedly disrupted lives. People were upset but not surprised that bad things happened.

Today with technology that helps us predict a good deal of the weather, prevents many diseases, air-conditions our homes and cars, takes us to the moon, etc., many of us have come to believe we can create a certain world and control it.

Unconsciously, we like to believe that technology can forestall bad events and when it doesn't, it's only because someone failed to take appropriate measures. We believe we can get back into control as soon as we discover whom to blame—and get rid of them. However, that doesn't work.

Paradoxically the great advances in technology, communications, transportation and growth of organizations have not improved our ability to predict outcomes. Often these advances create unintended and unwelcome consequences more difficult to foresee or to control. Simple examples of this increased complexity are more deadly terrorists, huge multi-national companies that no single government can regulate, a bacterium resistant to antibiotics, infants with special needs who would not have survived 20 years ago, and older, sicker patients who would have died in the hospitals of the 1980s, etc.

UNINTENDED CONSEQUENCES

All these changes demand new thinking to cope with the unintended consequences of complexity and new inventions occurring throughout society. Hospitals are the frontlines of this paradoxical change where good and bad effects need to be sorted, managed and improved. Systems thinking can do that.

The stories in this book are about managing —not controlling—an uncertain world and learning to predict outcomes and to produce what you intend.

AUTHORS

I am a journalist, and my co-author is a scholar. I produced an NBC documentary in 1980, **"If Japan Can...*Why Can't We?"*** It introduced systems thinking to the West and described how an American statistician, W. Edwards Deming, taught the Japanese to use it and work smarter not harder to produce continually improving automobiles and electronic goods. (**"If Japan Can..."** was named by **The Washington**

Times as the second most influential documentary in the history of motion pictures and television in 2005.)

It took me ten years to begin to understand this new mindset Dr. Deming was describing. That was in spite of the advantage of working with him the last 13 years of his life to explain these ideas in the 32-volume Deming Video Library. I gradually understood the many pieces of his philosophy, e.g. continual improvement, no blame or fear, cooperation rather than competition, etc. But even after I saw how groups or organizations of people working together with these rules and good leadership could be greater than the sum of their parts, it was difficult to explain. My breakthrough came when I videotaped a conversation between Dr. Deming and Dr. Russell Ackoff, Professor Emeritus at the University of Pennsylvania and author of seminal books on systems thinking. I finally understood that theirs was a different worldview of how to organize people and work to be more effective, efficient and personally rewarding.

In the late 1990s, I began to work with Dr. Louis M. Savary, a statistician, theologian and author, to study the systems mindset and how to teach it, particularly in the workplace. We concluded it can be most effectively communicated experientially, which is why we have written this book featuring the personal experiences of medical professionals as they learned systems thinking and began to apply it every day in hospitals.

WESTERN DIFFICULTIES

Systems thinking can be difficult for Americans and other Westerners. Western scientific thinking, which asks questions about the truth of the world and mounts experiments to test its theories, provides an essential element of systems thinking. However, it is only one element in the foundation or infrastructure of this revolutionary mindset.

Unlike the limited individualistic, single-focused, pragmatic, direct cause-and-effect approach of the scientific method, the systems mindset is about relatedness, interdependencies, and deep-seated causes. Instead of focusing on actions, it focuses on interactions—what happens between individuals and between teams, groups, and departments.

A system cannot be grasped by analysis, the backbone of scientific thinking. Analysis takes wholes, e.g., a machine, a piano, etc. apart and looks at the actions of the parts—how things work. In analysis the whole is equal to the sum of the parts. On the other hand, synthesis studies the interactions—why things happen. Systems thinking requires analysis and synthesis and the ability to appreciate a system's intangible and beyond-linear qualities, its greater whole, as well as the larger system of which it is a part. In synthesis, the whole is the product of the interactions of its parts. An easy example is a champion sports team, which is greater than the sum of its parts. Sadly most teams and organizations, even families or people, add up to less than the sum of their parts.

Experts have observed that this new way of thinking, the ability to grasp and appreciate a system, appears more attuned to Eastern philosophies of long-term cooperation, flow-of-life thinking and life-long learning than to Western principles of individualism, competition, quick fixes, and short-term results. Dr. Ackoff, America's leading system's teacher, says the East is learning scientific thinking more rapidly than the West is learning systems thinking. We think he is correct and that this is a serious problem for the West. Scientific thinking is easier for a systems thinker to learn than vice-versa.

This book is our effort to explain and help Americans reap the benefits of systems thinking as well as dramatically improve hospitals. When combined with scientific thinking, we believe it can produce an evolutionary leap in human consciousness and consequent effectiveness. That is beginning to happen in Pacific nations, which have a long history of appreciation for systems.

The West has been working with these ideas for more than 25 years. They have not been easy to explain or hold onto. For instance, the American automobile industry seemed to "get" them briefly in the early 1990s but soon lost them to a new generation of short-term-thinking managers and executives more interested in profit than pleasing customers.

DON'T BLAME HOSPITALS

It must be noted at the outset that not every hospital in the United States can be labeled "sick and dangerous." A number of American healthcare facilities have remarkably improved their organizational health. We are telling the particular how-to stories of these two large hospital groups. (And not incidentally, these hospitals are becoming more profitable as they improve services and reduce waste.)

Furthermore, we do not blame healthcare workers, hospitals or the people running them for the sorry state of healthcare delivery today. Today's hospital problems are the result of a nationwide healthcare management and delivery system that may have worked well enough in earlier times but is now overwhelmed by a complexity bordering on chaos. This complexity is intensified by a continuing avalanche of breakthroughs in technology, healthcare equipment and methods, a plethora of new drugs, sicker patients, a labyrinth of insurance reimbursement regulations, people living longer, reduced hospital stays, and a dramatic rise in chronic illnesses that hospitals are unprepared to treat. And this list does not factor in the millions of Americans without health insurance, many of whom could be served if health costs were reduced.

LEARNING TO WORK SMARTER NOT HARDER

This health system failure cannot be fixed by blaming individuals. Seeing and improving the system, rather than blaming individuals is a basic tenet of systems thinking.

At first glance, systems thinking sounds un-American. This is because many of the ideas and practices that made America great in simpler times not only don't work anymore, but now actually sabotage complex organizations like hospitals and schools.

For example, "doing your best," unless you understand how your work fits into the whole hospital, can make things worse. Nurses, who used to hide wheelchairs in a bathroom to save them for their patients, were doing their best to help make things better for those under their care. In a previous era, such nurses might have been seen as outstanding, caring employees with initiative. However, a story in the book explains how today in a large hospital complex, caring nurses stashing wheelchairs in bathrooms can help defeat the system. For example, such practices can spread diseases if the hidden chairs are not properly sanitized, cause a shortage of available wheelchairs, require new wheelchairs to be purchased, and delay many patients from getting the care they need.

Systems thinking also does away with blame and the American truism, "If it ain't broke, don't fix it." The foundation of systems thinking is improvement and cooperation, not competition. Its outlook is long-term, not short-term. Its focus is pleasing the customer/patient and finding effectiveness and joy in work. Systems thinking has also shown that, when used to focus on satisfying customers, company profits will take care of themselves.

In typical American linear logic, 2 + 2 always equals 4. In systems thinking, however, 2 + 2 may not only add up to four, but to 3 in a bad system, or to 22 in a great system. Any system can generate effects that are more—or less—than the sum of its parts. Showing people how to create a greater whole is the underlying purpose of systems thinking, i.e., getting more for less effort, working smarter not harder.

For a systems thinker, there is never a "best" way to do a job. Every process can always be improved. A systems thinker never stops learning and seeking ways to make something better.

ONE MORE THING

By the end of this book, you will know how a hospital or any organization can begin the process of transforming itself as well as how to identify a continually improving one. One American CEO of a major automobile corporation found the ideas of "never ending improvement" exhausting and depressing. We "can-do" Americans like to be finished with jobs and problems. That's not possible in continual improvement.

The readers we have in mind include healthcare consumers or potential patients, relatives of patients, hospital administrators, healthcare policy makers, hospital staff, physicians, healthcare insurers, employers paying for employee healthcare insurance, state and federal lawmakers, concerned taxpayers and people seeking to improve any organization.

Moreover, since everyone is a potential hospital patient, the issue of improving patient safety and care in our hospitals is vital to us all. Any one of us could be among those 200,000 patients who die each year in American hospitals, but don't have to.

Clare Crawford-Mason   *Louis M. Savary*

Washington, D.C.
April 2006

INTRODUCTION

The only consistent in health care is the anxious anticipation of change that never actually occurs.

J. D. Kleinke

A GOOD-NEWS STORY

A Google search of the topic "American hospitals + dangerous" produced a million and a half hits. More than five thousand books and published articles spell out how sick and dangerous many of today's hospitals really are. It's a bad-news story.

This book is different, for a number of reasons. Mostly, it's a good-news story.

- ◆ First, doctors, nurses and hospital administrators from two hospital groups freely talk about how sick their hospitals were, why they got sick, and how they learned to heal them.

- ◆ Second, these two healthcare systems healed themselves by using management principles taken from a most unlikely source—an auto manufacturer that uses systems thinking and quality methods.

- ◆ Third, while most efforts at organizational transformation fail after a short period, these two healthcare systems have achieved the transformation to organizational health and are maintaining it—one of them for over a decade—continually getting better and better.

- ◆ Fourth, they continue to maintain this transformation without outside help—they do it locally—without government assistance, expert consultants, new resources, new hires, or added expenses.

- ◆ Fifth, they continue to make improvements in patient satisfaction, employee satisfaction, significant reduction of waste in time and money, and, most importantly, reduction of hospital-induced patient infections, suffering, and death.

- ◆ Sixth, these healthcare systems are totally patient-focused, not doctor-focused or hospital-focused. Their nurses, doctors, administrators, and other employees are committed to delivering perfect patient care.

IX

◆ Seventh, this book is different because we let these savvy healthcare people tell their stories in their own words.

NOT ALL AUTO MANUFACTURERS ARE THE SAME

We said that these two healthcare systems healed themselves by using management principles taken from an auto manufacturer, but not all automakers are the same. Many American auto manufacturers view their organizations as huge machines, and see their employees, in many ways, as replaceable parts. This view is not helpful.

Toyota, the automaker whose principles were adopted by the healthcare systems we studied, views its organizations as complex social systems, where each employee learns to continually improve his or her work. Employees see making improvements as an integral part of their jobs.

G. Kenneth Turnbull, Ph.D., Executive Vice President of Alcoa, commenting on the application of Toyota principles to health care, explains why its systems were transferable to hospitals. The reason is that Toyota principles teach people how to improve work of any kind.

> The fact is that a patient is not a car, and never will be. So, if that were the problem we were trying to solve, we'd be stopped. However, the Toyota system is set up to identify customer needs in very clear ways, and to meet those needs in explicit, efficient, rapid, supplier-building methods. They're quite superior in the world of work, so if you said there was no work in health care, then we've got a gap. But as long as you confess that work's there, then I've got a solution.

What these hospital personnel gained from Toyota was the knowledge, training, and scientific tools to develop teams of people who could:

◆ become greater than the sum of their parts,

◆ work together more effectively and efficiently,

◆ continually improve the processes involved in their jobs,

◆ see how their individual work contributes to the aim of the whole system.

X

In this way, all employees in these hospitals become scientists, that is, they use scientific methods of experiment and testing to continually improve the work they do.

Any modern hospital can begin the process of self-healing if its doctors, nurses, aides, and administrators are universally committed to doing so. Once everyone is pledged to the singular purpose of achieving perfect patient care, they need to learn how to put on the new mindset—systems thinking—that will help them do the job.

Meet our two healthcare systems that have been succeeding.

SSM HEALTH CARE

SSM Health Care, headquartered in St. Louis, Missouri, is one of the largest Catholic healthcare systems in the United States. It owns, operates, and manages 23 facilities, including 20 acute care hospitals, in four states: Missouri, Wisconsin, Illinois and Oklahoma. SSM Health Care employs nearly 23,000 people and affiliates with approximately 5,000 physicians working in direct care facilities and related businesses.

During the 1980s like many other organizations and industries at the time, SSM Health Care developed a mission statement, identified its principles, and listed its key values. Part of that mission statement announced that they were committed to continually enhancing quality. They used a variety of conventional means to convey their mission, principles, and values. But for all their efforts and best intentions, as admitted in *CQI and the Renovation of an American Health Care System*, a book that tells the SSM story in great detail, they had "no operational structures or consistent management processes to ensure that their values were being acted on" daily in each facility. They wondered, in the words of their CEO, Sister Mary Jean Ryan, "What would it take to have the continual enhancement of quality simply be the way we work here?"

By 1989, SSM Health Care leadership had discovered the surprising link between quality theories used in manufacturing and how quality methods might be applied in health care. After all, Sister Mary Jean explains, "it does seem odd to refer to health care as a "product," the work of doctors and nurses as a "repeatable process," and patients as "customers."

But in making that connection, they began their process of self-healing. They hired the Process Management Institute to guide their executives through the principles and methods of quality theory and systems thinking, a version they called Continual Quality Improvement (CQI, for short). Within the year, they invited the entire SSM Health Care System to commit to a cultural revolution based on CQI principles.

During the mid-1990s, they began pursuing the prized Malcolm Baldrige National Quality Award. Studying the Baldrige criteria helped them to improve their processes and self-healing even more.

Senior Vice President in charge of strategic planning for SSM Health Care, William P. Thompson, described the early days this way:

> We started going through the Baldrige, using the Baldrige criteria as a framework for improvement. People said, "Sister, we don't have time to do the self-assessments. We don't have time to write the applications. We don't have time to do this. We have other crises, we have other problems, fires to fight, and everything else." And Sister has always listened to that input but has always relied on her own internal compass. She would say, "No, we are committed to this. I see enough improvement. It resonates with my personal values. I believe that this will help us become a better organization." And she has been the constant driver of this throughout the last 16 years at SSM Health Care.

In 2002, SSM Health Care was the first healthcare organization to receive the Malcolm Baldrige National Quality Award. Today, they continue to improve all their processes and systems in their unending desire to provide perfect patient care.

THE PITTSBURGH REGIONAL HEALTHCARE INITIATIVE (PRHI)

Our second good news story is about the Pittsburgh Regional Healthcare Initiative (PRHI), a collaborative effort including hundreds of clinicians, forty hospitals that compete for patients but cooperate to discover best practices, four major health insurers, dozens of major and small-business healthcare purchasers, corporate and civic leaders, and Pennsylvania's attorney general. It forms a unique collaborative effort of individuals and institutions that provide, purchase, insure and support healthcare services throughout Southwestern Pennsylvania.

XII

PRHI Chair & Founder, Karen Wolk Feinstein, explains its origins and inspiration.

> The issue at the time was the cost of health care. We wanted to draw attention to the fact that we thought regions didn't have to wait for a national solution to the increasing costs of health care but could fashion a solution locally within their own region.

It should be noted that healthcare delivery is that region's largest single industry and shapes the life of each member of the community, as of course it does in other communities.

Raymond LeBoeuf, CEO of PPG Industries, a major employer in the Pittsburgh area, added,

> We discovered as a community, both public and private, that health care was chewing into to our total level of resources. Our pie is only so big, and if the health care piece of that pie gets greater and greater, other things will shrink and that does not auger well for Pittsburgh.

The members of PRHI are working together to achieve "the world's best patient outcomes" by continually improving health system performance by identifying and solving problems at the point of patient care. They believe that the many challenges facing health care today—rising costs, overcapacity, frustration among clinicians, shortage of workers, financial distress, malpractice crisis, and lack of access to care—are all symptoms of the same root problem: failure of the system to focus solely on patient needs.

Like SSM Health Care in St. Louis, the Pittsburgh Regional Healthcare Initiative used systems-thinking principles and continual quality improvement methods in order to achieve their needed transformation. PRHI turned to the Toyota Production System.

Paul O'Neill, former U.S. Treasury Secretary and former CEO of PRHI, was previously CEO of Alcoa, where he used Toyota methods to deliver an 800 percent increase in market capitalization while making it one of the safest companies in the world to work for. He emphasized the pioneering quality of PRHI's efforts:

> For me, this is a really an important step, one of many we need to take in Pittsburgh, to demonstrate to the rest of the country

and the rest of the world that we don't have to take what we have as a given and accept medication errors and infections that are acquired in the hospital that you didn't bring with you and in being given incorrect procedures that stem from a lack of knowledge or training.

In light of healthcare statistics across the country, some of their patient-centered goals—zero medication errors, zero hospital-acquired infections, and perfect clinical results as measured by complications, readmissions and other patient outcomes—seem impossible to attain. But they are committed to work toward these goals. This book explains why this pursuit of perfection in health care is inspiring and effective. And, meanwhile, within three months of real-time problem solving in one area of the intensive care unit, the number of hospital-acquired infections was reduced to zero and has remained at zero.

A SPIRIT OF HOPE AND OPTIMISM

In the following pages, doctors, nurses, aides, and administrators tell how and why these two healthcare systems are getting better at making patients safer and safer.

They talk about their amazement at seeing their own work with new eyes, the satisfaction of learning how to organize things more effectively, their delight at improved medical outcomes and happier patients, and their surprise at how much more they are enjoying their work.

Physicians tell how being fully involved in their hospital's self-healing can give new life to their medical careers. Nurses testify that their hospital's self-healing gives them the chance to be truly nurses again.

Administrators tell how they learned to manage healthcare facilities that are growing healthier and more patient-centered every day.

Instead of describing only the sickness of hospitals and how dangerous they continue to be, this book is meant to inspire hope and optimism. In its chapters the personnel describe in their own words the organizational cure and how hospitals can become patient-centered.

The book is divided into three parts. People from SSM Health Care and PRHI tell, first, about the problems they faced, second, the solutions they found and, third, the path of their improvement.

PART I:

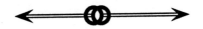

Problems

CHAPTER 1

WHERE WE STARTED:
SYMPTOMS OF SICK HOSPITALS

Americans are accustomed to getting every day mir-
acles out of the healthcare system to keep us alive and
well, well past what our parents or grandparents could
have ever imagined. But the system that delivers those
miracles is also rife with waste and inefficiency to an
extent that I think very few Americans appreciate.

Cliff Shannon, President, SMC Business Council,
Pittsburgh, PA

THE LONG LIST OF SYMPTOMS

There are a surprising number of problems or symptoms in hospitals in need of healing: astounding waste, dissatisfied patients, unnecessary duplication of costly services among neighboring hospitals (e.g., helicopters and expensive diagnostic machinery), medication errors, medical errors, deadly infections the hospital gives the patient, worker safety, high death rates from errors, overcrowded emergency rooms, lack of standardized performance steps for many procedures, lack of coordination of patient care, long waits, multiplication of expensive tests to forestall lawsuits, conflicting incentives from insurance companies for hospitals and doctors.

It is a long and troubling list, but it is vitally important to understand that these symptoms do not cast blame on individual healthcare workers or individual hospitals. They can be attributed to a faulty system that has evolved in modern industrial countries as healthcare delivery has changed. Ironically, as health care has gotten better—new drugs, procedures, technology and knowledge—the delivery of health care has become worse. The way many of today's hospital processes and procedures have evolved almost prohibits adequate patient-centered care. These hospitals just grew as new advances, changes and regulations were absorbed with little thought or time to consider ef-

1

fectiveness or efficiency. To make matters worse, the complex, modern patient is generally older and sicker than the patients of the past because of advances in medicine.

The respected Institute of Medicine reported on the quality of American health care in *Crossing the Quality Chasm: A New Health System for the 21st Century*. It did not paint a rosy picture. The authors began their report,

> The frustration levels of both patients and clinicians have probably never been higher. Yet the problem remains. Health care today harms too frequently and routinely fails to deliver its potential benefits. [1]

The doctors, nurses, administrators and other staff at PRHI and SSM Health Care understood this challenge when they began to try to improve their hospitals. They first formally recognized that their hospitals needed improvement, which is the first step in any improvement program. This is unusually difficult for medical workers because they are dealing in human life and suffering and are dedicated to helping people. However, they discovered the symptoms were evident and alarming, particularly serious patient safety issues.

> I felt as if much of what I did didn't matter. I had good relationships with my patients but my ability to really affect their overall outcome was somewhat limited. So, like many physicians today, I felt powerless. I felt embroiled in issues surrounding medical legal matters such as the malpractice crisis. I was overwhelmed with the requirements of what payers in my institution wanted in terms of my documentations. I felt as if I was being further and further removed from the bedside. And I thought it was probably time for a change.
>
> *Richard Shannon, MD, Chairman, Department of Medicine,*
> *Allegheny General Hospital, PRHI*

> It's a system that's producing defects, errors, patient death, patient injuries and other forms of less than optimum care at a rate that is almost beyond imagination. The way that health

care is delivered in just about every hospital in the country is well close to being insane.

Cliff Shannon, President, SMC Business Council,
Pittsburgh, PA

There certainly have been gaps identified in the quality of health care, in the reliability of health care, in the safety of health care, and certainly in the unaffordability of health care both to individual patients as well as to the nation as a whole. These are certainly issues we face.

Andrew Kosseff, MD, Director,
Clinical Systems Improvement, SSM Health Care

Studies suggest that, each year in the United States, at least two million hospital patients get dangerous infections and diseases they didn't come with, and well over 100,000 die from them. These are infections they acquired in the hospital, often airborne or transmitted by hand; that is, patients get infected when a physician or staff person moves from tending one patient to another without disinfecting their hands. These hospital-acquired infections have become so prevalent—growing in number and virulence—in modern hospitals that they have been given a special name.

Nosocomial is a very interesting word. It didn't exist a few decades ago. It was invented by the healthcare community to sort of camouflage what it really means, which is "hospital-acquired." So, a hospital-acquired infection is now referred to as a nosocomial infection. The very fact that you have to ask what a nosocomial infection is, is testament to how effective that camouflage is.

Peter Perreiah, Director,
Pittsburgh Regional Healthcare Initiative

Infections are just one issue.

Too many people have to return to the hospital too many times for the same illness. Too many people wait endless hours to get an appointment or to be seen in the emergency room, or to be seen anyplace. And then when they do finally get treatment, they are not satisfied with it because of the way that they've been treated—without dignity, without respect, and in a hurry. And many times they haven't really been treated at all. They have gone through a whole series of tests—to some great discomfort, I might add—only to find out that very often they are not correctly diagnosed.

Sister Mary Jean Ryan, FSM, RN, President & CEO,
SSM Health Care

In addition to the serious harm inflected on patients, there is also waste and inefficiency.

If you have people sitting in an emergency room waiting for emergency care for five, six, seven, eight hours—sometimes twelve hours—that's a sign of a sick hospital. If you have patients that are being admitted to the hospital sitting in the emergency department waiting for a bed for 12, 24, 48 hours, that's a sign of a sick hospital.

Tim Thompson, DO, Emergency Room Director,
SSM St Joseph's Hospital West

Another symptom is what hospital professionals call layering:

Physicians aren't typically trained in systems management, so when a problem occurs, instead of fixing the root cause of the problem, we add one more layer of things to do. Instead of going back to root cause, we'll work around this problem or work around this person who isn't doing his or her job correctly. We'll work around everything. When you do that a hundred times on a hospital floor over a span of a decade, pretty soon no one can remember why they are doing anything the way they do it. To add one more layer to things you're already doing provides no logical progress from the thing that you're trying to do—caring for a patient—to the things that the staff who are involved in healthcare delivery are doing and are often required to do.

Cliff Shannon, President, SMC Business Council,
Pittsburgh, PA

We've overlaid one system on top of another system on top of another system, and we've made a lot of decisions away from the front line of the patient. I think what has happened is the care systems have gotten so badly broken, it makes it very hard for people to do the right thing.

Deborah Thompson, RN, Quality Trainer,
PRHI

When a new regulation comes into play that we need to incorporate into our business, we tend to add that new regulation without taking a step back and asking ourselves, "Okay, what do we need to do from this point on differently than we've done before?"

Maggie Fowler, Vice President of Patient Services
SSM St. Joseph's Health Center

There is so much duplication in health care, and the need for coordination among healthcare providers is so prevalent today.

Paula Friedman, Vice President, Systems Improvement,
SSM Health Care

It's been layered on for so long. Different things got layered on that maybe had a rationale or a reason when they were layered on, and they became standard behavior. But even though such behaviors long ago lost their reasoning, people still keep doing them. There are some things that no one could ever explain to you why they are still being done this way. It's dysfunctional.

Karen Wolk Feinstein, Chair & Founder, PRHI
President, Jewish Healthcare Foundation

A lot of what we have developed is a very complicated process of care, which sometimes, ironically, not only adds cost to the care but also can add potential injury to the patient.

William Schoenhard, Executive VP & COO,
SSM Health Care

All the experts seem to agree that quality problems in hospitals occur typically not because of a lack of good will, best intentions, knowledge, effort, equipment, money or other resources devoted to health care, but because of fundamental shortcomings in the ways care is or-

5

ganized. Today's hospital systems often lack the strategy, the leadership, the environment, the policies, the processes, and the capabilities necessary to guarantee that the services patients receive are safe, effective, efficient, and equitable.

Again, this is not because people who manage or work in hospitals are bad or not smart. Managing and working in a modern complex delivery system isn't easy as American auto manufacturers have finally and sadly discovered. There has been more change in the last century than all preceding centuries. Learning to anticipate, accept and manage change is complex and difficult. Most traditional management systems were not designed to deal with rapid and complex changes.

The primary and most important symptom of sick hospitals is not easy to describe or diagnose, because it is a missing method of managing the hospital. It is when the hospital leaders and workers do not know how to view the hospital as a whole system, and organize or re-organize their work to continually improve the delivery of health care. Continual improvement will always reduce costs. A hospital is a complicated, high-tech, but hands-on enterprise and the workers have too little hard information or modern management methods to identify best practices or the most effective way to make the hospital safer and more effective and efficient. The work and the demand for documentation become more and more complex every day.

The variety of preceding comments—from a number of hospitals across the country and all levels in healthcare—illustrate that sick hospitals are a national problem. Each person's testimony builds a more critical case for addressing this increasingly deadly situation. In the following chapters, people from PRHI and SSM Health Care tell about their biggest challenge, their most surprising challenge, and their most pervasive challenge.

SOME THINGS TO REMEMBER FROM THIS CHAPTER

✓ Because American medicine has cured so many more illnesses and physical conditions over the past 40 or 50 years, many people tend to overlook how sick hospitals are.

✓ Hospital staff do their best, but that is no longer effective to manage the rapidly changing, complex healthcare delivery system.

✓ The medical staff knows conditions are worsening, but it is not clear what to do. The sick hospital diagnosis is not about bad people but a broken system that needs new management practices.

✓ The first step toward healing hospitals is to begin to recognize, describe and discuss the problem.

✓ The legal, profit-driven and blame aspects of American society make this step painful and difficult.

CHAPTER FOOTNOTES

[1] Institute of Medicine (2001) *Crossing the Quality Chasm: A New Health System for the 21st Century*. Washington, DC: National Academy of Sciences, page 1.

CHAPTER 2

THE BIGGEST CHALLENGE WE FACED: COMPLEXITY

It's a very slow process, reforming health care delivery. In my experience it is the most complex production system and delivery of service system that exists in the world. Maybe there is some highly sophisticated weapons system that in some aspect is that complex, or more so, but I haven't heard of it.

Cliff Shannon, President, SMC Business Council,
Pittsburgh, PA

OVERALL COMPLEXITY OF THE HEALTHCARE SYSTEM

Hospitals today are huge and constantly changing. Today's hospital problems are the result of a nationwide healthcare delivery system that worked well enough in earlier times but now is overwhelmed by a complexity near chaos. This complexity is generated by a continuing flood of breakthroughs in technology, healthcare equipment and methods, a myriad of new drugs on the market, sicker patients, a maze of insurance reimbursement regulations, people living longer with new and more serious diseases and at the same time reduced hospital stays, and a dramatic rise in chronic illnesses, which hospitals are unprepared to treat.

The amount of complexity has increased both in technology, medications available, treatments, payment mechanisms, and in the ability of physicians and patients to interact and to relate.

Paul Convery, MD, Chief Medical Officer
SSM Health Care/St. Louis

When you had a heart attack 22 years ago, your only choice was bypass surgery, and that was still a relatively new technique. Today, we can offer you not only a regular stent but we can offer you a drug-coated stent. We can offer you a full cabg (Coronary artery bypass graft); we can offer you a mini cabg. We don't have to harvest your leg vein any more. We can offer you cadaver veins. I mean the options that are available to a patient today are easily ten times more than what they were 22 years ago.

Tami Merryman, RN, Vice President, Patient Care Services,
Shadyside Hospital, PRHI

MORE COMPLEX TREATMENTS

Historically, treatments of specific illnesses were limited and in some sense straight-forward, even if outcomes were not as favorable as today. With a dramatic increase in treatment options, clinical results may be improved, but the coordination among the health care providers to manage these medicines and procedures has not kept pace. Our two hospital systems clearly address these issues by adopting a system of management that has continual improvement built in.

I think that one of the greatest things that have changed in medicine and practice is how sick people have become and how complex the treatments that they need, required to be performed by nurses and other allied health professionals.

You know, it used to be you'd come into one department; you'd have one test. We'd figure out what was wrong with you and we'd send you home. Pretty simple process. Now, you come into the hospital and you might need to visit 25 departments to have 30 different diagnostic tests that all need to be integrated and coordinated. And multiple specialists are involved in making the decisions about your treatment plans. Yet the management systems are still somewhat geared to the past.

Tami Merryman, RN, Vice President, Patient Care Services,
Shadyside Hospital, PRHI

You may come in to have a surgical procedure and go home the same day, so that's really changed. How we are able to treat and manage many diseases has changed. And the intensity of care delivered to patients is much greater.

Tim Thompson, DO, Emergency Room Director,
SSM St Joseph's Hospital West

The use of hospitals, specialties, different diagnostic techniques, these have all increased the complexity. And as you increase the complexity of the system and the organization and as you increase the complexity of the relationships, you just increase the potential for errors and misadventures.

Paul Convery, MD, Chief Medical Officer,
SSM Health Care/St. Louis

There have been explosions in technology and biotechnology that have been able to help a lot of patients to lead much better lives and have also added a great deal of complication as to how care can be provided to patients.

Dennis Schilling, Clinical Coordinator,
PRHI

PATIENTS ARE SICKER AND HAVE MORE COMPLEX PROBLEMS

Because of all the advances in medicine, many patients alive today would have died in the past. So the patients are sicker and have more complex diseases, but insurance payers require that hospital stays be shorter.

Today, people are more ill in some situations, and that's a real challenge because the length of stay in hospitals is shorter than it has been in the past.

Eunice Halverson, Corporate Vice President,
Quality Resource Center, SSM Health Care

Patients are more complex and lengths of stay are shorter, so we have sicker patients and less time to take care of them. Their drug utilization expense is higher because we are using fancier things up front so we can send them home faster. But then they return because what we did wasn't quite enough or we did not allow enough time to make sure that they were safe and stable to go to the next level of care. There are a lot of questions that aren't answered yet.

Kelley A. Wasicek, R.Ph., Pharmacy Manager,
UPMC Presbyterian Hospital, PRHI

In (the past), a lot of our patients were not as sick as they are today. We had a lot of patients then. I might have twenty patients on my side of the unit, and it could be that seven to ten of them might be up and about, who could have taken care of themselves. That just doesn't happen today. Hardly anybody is up and about today unless nurses are walking them in the hall after surgery or recovery from something.

Sister Mary Jean Ryan, FSM, RN, President & CEO,
SSM Health Care

We've extended people's lives. We've extended lives so that people who have compromised life styles actually utilize the hospital more. We see many more patients with end stage renal disease than we used to. We see heart transplant patients or other organ transplant patients, and these folks ultimately get into trouble that I never saw when I was a medical student.

Filippo Ferrigni, MD, VP, Critical Care Director
SSM St. Joseph's Health Center

Higher Expectations

It is not only doctors who are better educated. Patients today have more knowledge and higher expectations

Perhaps one of the most significant advances we've seen is the increased expectations of patients. When I first started years ago, patients came into the hospital and would accept anything we did to them. I think, as the U.S. society has...higher expectations of all those who provide service to them, that expectation is happening in health care.

Chris Grass, Clinical Pharmacist,
SSM DePaul Health Center

11

Health care is a lot better today than it was 30 or 40 years ago. We know a lot more today. The doctors are very much better educated and their specialties abound. What people had forty years ago were simple questions and simple answers, with people expecting a limited amount of help and doctors then met their requirements.

Raymond LeBoeuf, CEO, PPG Industries,
Pittsburgh, PA

People are more aware of their conditions, symptoms, and illnesses, and how to treat them. There's an onslaught of advertisements on television. People are starting to self diagnose more. We have the internet where people get a lot of information about taking care of themselves, and they go to the doctors more or less demanding "this medication that I read about in the magazine" or saw advertised on television or looked up on the internet. So we see a lot more interest in self-care and self-diagnosis

Chris Grass, Clinical Pharmacist,
SSM DePaul Health Center

Hospitals Have Become a Big Complex Business

And all the complexity and cost have turned what were small institutions for mostly simple operations and palliative care into huge buildings offering many complicated treatments—in other words, into big businesses.

I think the big, big shift is really that health care has become big business, and it's become difficult business.

Kevin Johnson, MD, VP for Medical Affairs,
SSM DePaul Health Center

Insurance companies require increased paper work and documentation, which has had a large impact on the efficient way or lack thereof in delivering medicine and the amount of time it takes to ensure that you take care of someone correctly for reimbursement.

William P. Thompson, Senior Vice President,
Strategic Development, SSM Health Care

In the Pittsburgh region, a doctor's office receives information from four different commercial health plans, three different Medicaid plans, Medicare and dozens of labs in the area. The fax machine is whirring all day; lab reports are constantly coming in. These get put in the "to be filed" stack, which doesn't necessarily mean it will be the order in which they are taken care of, and the way they are sorted doesn't necessarily mean they will be available when a patient comes in to be seen. That the information for that patient is in the file at the hour that the patient comes in to the doctor's office happens very rarely.

Tania Lyon, Ph.D., Chronic Care Coordinator,
PRHI

ARCHAIC MANAGEMENT PRACTICES

Effective and efficient management practices—or ways to organize people to produce continually improving healthcare services—have not kept pace with the increased and complex services offered. The key people—doctors and nurses—received medical educations and relatively few were interested in or pursued learning about the rapidly changing theories for managing complex organizations such as modern hospitals. In the 20th Century, hospital administration was generally an intuitive, seat-of-the-pants operation, which worked until expensive technological and pharmaceutical advances and a climate of continual new regulations made health service delivery exponentially complicated.

We have 50, 60, 70 years of tradition, history, experience, practice that we have to overcome.

William P. Thompson, Senior Vice President,
Strategic Development, SSM Health Care

We are really now beginning to understand that we have archaic processes in our hospitals that for the most part set up our clinicians in an atmosphere that allows them to make errors.

JoAnn V. Narduzzi, MD, Vice President, Academic Affairs,
Pittsburgh Mercy Health System, PRHI

At PRHI we know from the Robert Wood Johnson Foundation study that there is a 17-year lag between the publication of a piece of medical knowledge about best practice for a medical problem and the time when it becomes generally accepted as medical practice.

Tania Lyon, Ph.D., Chronic Care Coordinator,
PRHI

To further compound problems there is a conflict in incentives between doctors and hospitals.

If you're an internist and you have a patient admitted with a myocardial infarction the hospital gets paid a fixed payment, whether you stay one day, two days, five days. But if you're a physician, you get paid daily. So your incentive is to keep the patient longer. The hospital's incentive is to get the patient out. And it's just the beginning of the first conflicts between the doctor's needs and the hospital's needs.

JoAnn V. Narduzzi, MD, Ph.D., VP of Academic Affairs,
Pittsburgh Mercy Health System, PRHI

NOT A KNOWLEDGE GAP, BUT OVERWHELMING COMPLEXITY

So it's not a knowledge gap. It's not that we don't have physicians and nurses that are smart and know this. But the complexities of taking care of the patients can be so overwhelming. There are so many things going on at the same time. There are so many different demands that it's really beyond the capability of even very bright, well-intentioned people to remember every single detail. And so you have to build a system that reminds them of the detail or alerts them to ordering the aspirin and beta-blocker. You still leave it up to the physician or the nurse to make the clinical decisions, but you need to have that alert or that reminder built into the system

Paul Convery, MD, Chief Medical Officer
SSM Health Care/St. Louis

Since medical knowledge is not the problem, part of the solution begins to take form: a failsafe system of standardized practices based on sound data will work in many cases.

We have over 30 order sets for the common diseases, which bring structure to that treatment plan to try and prevent folks— really very good and talented people—from making simple errors of oversight... It's dotting the i's and crossing the t's that saves a great number of lives in the hospital. Most people have common diseases for which we have common and very effective treatments.

Filippo Ferrigni, MD, VP, Critical Care Director,
SSM St. Joseph's Health Center

A fail-safe system is not as difficult or Utopian as it sounds. The first vital step in creating a fail-safe system is identifying and describing the problems and challenges so the system can be designed. That is why this book begins by discussing the problems of hospitals. And even this necessary first step is not easily accomplished in hospitals these days.

A DESPERATE NEED FOR SYSTEMS THINKING

In most of today's hospitals, administrators continue, often fruitlessly, to apply traditional management tools that are no longer adequate to control the tumultuous complexity and contemporary chaos overpowering their facilities.

Almost all of those no-longer-useful management tools were based on linear reasoning and single-event thinking, a mindset designed for running an organization during a much simpler era than ours. Everyone is familiar with typical methods of that traditional system: management by objectives, putting out "fires" as they occur, making little fixes here and there whenever a problem emerged, or "if it ain't broke, don't fix it," adding more security, duplicating services, doubling and tripling inspection personnel, putting up posters, hiring flavor-of-the-month consultants, buying the latest equipment, giving motivational exhortations, passing the buck, offering incentives—or threats, and blaming. The list of those we tend to blame is quite large. It includes government regulations, labor unions, insurers increased prices, paperwork, poor training, lack of skilled professionals, malpractice actions, laziness, etc., etc.

The two hospital systems we studied experienced all of these complexities and were being overwhelmed by them. Only later, as we describe in Part II, when they had begun to master systems thinking and the systems perspective it could provide, would they be able to see the big picture, create a new culture, learn to manage the necessary conversion of their systems and processes, and begin healing their hospitals.

While complexity might be the biggest challenge these hospitals faced, their most surprising discovery was the "lost patient." Complexity, one might say, made it difficult to "see" the patient. We will see how systems thinking helped them rediscover the patient. We look at the "missing" patient next.

SOME THINGS TO REMEMBER FROM THIS CHAPTER

✓ Hospitals have become more complex and will continue to become more complex.

✓ Traditional management approaches are overwhelmed by complexity; what is needed is a management that can handle continual change.

✓ The problem is not medical but managerial.

✓ Systems thinking is the solution.

✓ Systems thinking, remember, teaches people to recognize answers in terms of better processes and problems as faulty processes.

CHAPTER 3

THE MOST SURPRISING
CHALLENGE WE FACED:
THE LOST PATIENT

*Before, we nurses would put patients to bed at night.
We would give them a back rub. We would straighten
up the room. We would take the newspapers out. We
would prepare them very carefully.*

*Sister Mary Jean Ryan, FSM, RN, President & CEO,
SSM Health Care*

A UNIFYING PURPOSE

Anyone familiar with systems thinking or Dr. W. Edwards Deming's principles of quality management will know that the only thing that can turn a collection of people and machines into a true system, that is, make them a whole greater than the sum of their parts, is a *shared purpose.*

According to the theory, once you get everyone on board, committed to the same aim or purpose, you have created a basic system. Without that shared commitment, a group of people, even if they are working side by side in the same organization, do not enjoy a unified energy nor understanding of their task. There are simply many energies going in many directions, frequently at cross purposes. *A group's shared aim or purpose is their unifying force.* Nothing less could possibly unify them.

It is startling to realize how few organizations have a single shared aim or purpose. For example, in many hospitals each department has developed its own aim or purpose independent of others. Typically, in a hospital, the purchasing department's aim may be to save money; the administration's aim may be to make a profit and ensure the hospital's conformity to layers of government regulations; the aim in operating rooms may be to complete surgeries successfully; accounting's aim may be to maximize income from patients and their insurers; nursing's purpose may be to see that the patients on their unit are looked after. In the end, what you observe is the energies of many people going in many different directions and frequently in conflict and at cross-purposes. The unacknowledged cross-purposes are one of the first problems to be acknowledged in beginning to heal the hospital.

In contrast, the Toyota organization has a single purpose—to build cars with the highest quality that satisfy and delight customers. This purpose permeates every department in every Toyota plant and every Toyota employee. All their energies move in one direction, toward a single purpose.

Dr. Deming, who worked with Toyota in its early days, would say that, no matter what products or services your organization may provide, the only possible unifying purpose for that organization to pursue must be *to satisfy and even delight each customer*. If it weren't for the customers, he reminds us, there would be no need for that organization. Customers are any organization's reason for being.

In a hospital or any healthcare facility, the customer who needs to be satisfied and delighted is, of course, the *patient*. This truth is so obvious that it's astounding that so many in health care have missed it. If it weren't for the patients, there would be no need for their hospitals.

Among the hospitals we studied for this book, the most crucial awareness they developed was that, amid all the complexity and rapid changes happening in health care, they had, paradoxically, "forgotten" or "lost" the patient.

The biggest lesson they learned from their training in systems thinking and the Toyota Production System was that, until they made the patient's needs and patient care their unifying purpose, they would never become a true system.

Furthermore, they realized that only with an aim or purpose like "providing perfect patient care" could they begin to measure their organization's healing or know when it was improving.

So, they each made the giant step from losing sight of the patient to making perfect patient care *the* reason for their existence as a healthcare system.

IDENTIFYING THE PROBLEM

The patient began to fade from the hospital radar about 20 to 30 years ago. Until that time, healthcare workers couldn't do too much for the patient from back rubs to house calls.

But as complexity increased the organization of hospitals changed. Health care lost its focus on the patient and became focused on its own bureaucracy and policy mechanisms. Most hospitals today are designed around the needs of doctors, nurses, and hospital administrators and almost everyone is overburdened by paperwork required by insurers and governmental regulations

> It's very clear when you sit at the patient's bedside that the patient is not the customer, that the enterprise isn't organized around the patient. The patient is not the organizing principle for health care. It is so apparent.
>
> *Karen Wolk Feinstein, Chair & Founder, PRHI,*
> *President, Jewish Healthcare Foundation*

> In many cases I believe the patient has been kind of forgotten about, even though it doesn't seem like that makes a lot of sense. I really believe that's happened.
>
> *Marty Kurth, RN, Hospital Quality Trainer,*
> *PRHI*

> You come in and register in a hospital. You wait, you wait, and you wait in a doctor's office. Physicians are late, you wait for services, and you have to go through a managed care to get pre-certification or a referral to get anything done.
>
> *JoAnn V. Narduzzi, MD, Ph.D., VP of Academic Affairs,*
> *Pittsburgh Mercy Health System, PRHI*

> Well, in today's traditional hospital the nurses and the doctors and the policies and procedures are set up to make their work flow easier, I believe, and sometimes that doesn't fit with the needs of the patients.
>
> *Eunice Halverson, Corporate Vice President,*
> *Quality Resource Center, SSM Health Care*

What's so odd is that you can go into a video store and they have a record of every video that you've rented for the last nine years and every transaction. But you go and register at a hospital and, many times, most hospitals don't know that you were there yesterday. You have to re-give all of the same information.

Paula Friedman, Vice President, Systems Improvement,
SSM Health Care

HOW THE PATIENT GOT LOST

The loss of focus on the patient happened gradually, due to the circumstances of the complexity problems outlined in Chapter 2. This shift was not intentional, but because hospitals did not, in general, take a strategic view of their institution, they did not ask how a new technology or external requirement would affect the staff and the overall healthcare delivery system. They simply added the new technology or requirement to the current functioning of the hospital, without looking at how the work would now be accomplished and whether a reorganization of departments, or work processes, was needed to do a better job. Adding new technology or requirements to a hospital is like the build-up of barnacles on the hull of a ship over time. Also, now that multiple doctors are involved in the care of each patient, coordination and integration become more difficult.

The patient got lost amidst the growing complexity of the health care system.

Kenneth Segel, former Executive Director,
PRHI

We've overlaid one system on top of another system and another system, and we've made a lot of decisions away from the front line of the patient.

Deborah Thompson, RN, Quality Trainer,
PRHI

20

I made house calls up through the 1980's. I think the patient probably got lost somewhere in the process of large hospitals, managed care, the focus on insurance and benefits, and most recently in the emphasis on intense medical specialization—as opposed to focusing on patients and a patient's outcome.

Paul Convery, MD, Chief Medical Officer,
SSM Health Care/St. Louis

The average primary care physician is now scheduling office visits 12 minutes apart. That's how frequently patients are coming into a doctor's office. There's not enough time for a doctor to assess how a patient is doing and have a meaningful conversation or to do ongoing education.

Tania Lyon, Ph.D., Chronic Care Coordinator,
PRHI

THE DOWNSIDE OF TECHNOLOGY

While medical technology has clearly aided in extending people's lives, these advancements have their downsides. Technology, whether it is medical or informational, needs to be integrated with people's needs. Technology is only useful if it contributes to the efficiency and effectiveness of institutions as judged by the "customer," or patient in the case of a hospital.

Obviously technology has really blossomed, and there's a good side and a bad side to that. The good side is that we have many, many more opportunities to identify diseases, to assess patients, and to cure people or to help people. The downside is, I think, people are living longer than they used to and maybe not in the most ideal state of health. We may be keeping people alive too long in some situations, and technology, I think, has done that. There is a reliance on technology and sometimes we may rely on it too much, and then we lose that touch—because the human touch is so important.

Eunice Halverson, Corporate Vice President,
Quality Resource Center, SSM Health Care

THE ANSWER: PATIENT FOCUS

The focus on making the patient's needs the aim of a hospital is not as simple as the concept sounds. This does not mean that if every staff member were to think about the patient at every decision point, the medical outcomes would be better and hospitals would run more efficiently. That is because the complexities and interdependencies of the overlay of systems almost ensure that improving or changing one individual's work process may have a negative impact on the larger system.

The leaders began to ask new questions and see how departmental barriers were making patient care more complex and less effective.

> We have built up a bureaucracy in health care that is truly focused on the bureaucracy. We are doing things for the benefit of ourselves. We are designed to provide care in silos and fragments, fragments within a hospital. We have fragmentation between the hospital and the physician, and fragmentation between the hospital, physician and other providers. We have to break those barriers down and truly come together as a team, with the patient as our primary focus, and ask ourselves how we can best take care of this patient. How can we insure they get the preventive maintenance, the acute care, and the primary care when they need it? How do we do that in a way that it disrupts the patients' lives as minimally as possible?
>
> *William P. Thompson, Senior Vice President,*
> *Strategic Development, SSM Health Care*

Focusing on the patient's needs and safety is even more important and logical than it appears. For a complex technical and social system such as a hospital to work, everyone in the system—healthcare workers, administrators, support staff, insurance companies, employers providing insurance—must have a common aim: the health of the patient. That aim cannot be simply to reduce costs. That will happen automatically as the entire hospital system is understood and realigned to address patient needs.

Work is redesigned and re-organized with an understanding of how each department and healthcare staff member affects perfect patient care. Everyone in the healthcare system—inside and outside the hospital—must commit to the aim of the system: continually improving patient care.

> It's a critical challenge to keep the idea of the patient foremost. It's about the patient. It's about the person. It's about what we're always trying to do. It's easy to get lost in the details around that.
>
> *Kenneth Segel, former Executive Director,*
> *PRHI*

> I think that refocusing on the patient and what the patient needs is a very powerful tool in our regional initiative to get people thinking back where medicine is supposed to start. It's very easy for people to get distracted in the issues of finance or in hospital politics or in competition between each other. When we've been able to refocus people on the goal of the whole endeavor—getting the best possible patient outcomes—people really come together and collaborate to do the best they can to improve patient care. And they share information in the best possible ways.
>
> *Geoff Webster, Associate Director,*
> *PRHI*

The patient must commit as well. To involve patients in their care, both hospital systems are dedicated to patient education for prevention of disease and for follow-up care.

> Patients need to be their own doctors in a sense. Certainly there's no physician who can manage diabetes as well as a patient who is motivated and interested in controlling their own blood sugar because they're only going to see the doctor once a month. They're going to be their own doctor 31 days a month. And I think that's really important.
>
> *Filippo Ferrigni, MD, VP, Critical Care Director,*
> *SSM St. Joseph's Health Center*

Another important point in improving healthcare delivery is identifying waste. As we said earlier, systems management reduces costs and shows the way to more efficient and effective services. That's the next chapter.

Some Things to Remember From This Chapter

✓ The good news and the bad news turned out to be the same, the lost patient.

✓ No one had intended to overlook the patient but the downside of the amazing new technology and pharmaceuticals that saved more lives, etc., was complexity and distraction from the traditional person-to-person practice of medicine.

✓ The good news was that noticing how the patient had slipped off the radar gave the entire hospital system a new, mutual, and invigorating aim: everyone could agree on improved patient care and safety, even the insurance companies.

✓ A system must have an aim and a system must be managed. Making the patient the focus of everyone in the system makes it much easier to see the system, sort through the complexity (Chapter 2) and symptoms of a sick hospital (Chapter 1) and began to move toward healing the hospital.

CHAPTER 4

THE MOST PERVASIVE CHALLENGE WE FACED: WASTE

It is estimated that there is up to 40 percent waste in the U.S. healthcare system. That is, services are provided that aren't necessary, visits that aren't necessary, utilizing of higher levels of acuity that aren't necessary, for example, using acute care when out-patient care would be satisfactory, or seeing a physician where seeing a physician's assistant would be satisfactory. Ordering tests that aren't used for treatment. Unnecessary procedures.

William P. Thompson, Senior Vice President,
Strategic Development, SSM Health Care

A PROBLEM WITH A SOLUTION

Waste is a big problem for all organizations, so it is not surprising to hear hospital administrators bemoan the amount of waste they see around them. Waste generates higher costs, it eats away at profits, it cripples attempts at improvement, makes work more complicated and less effective, it sucks energy and enthusiasm out of people, and can sabotage success.

Some of the most common forms waste takes in organizations include gathering useless information, duplication of efforts, repetition of services, rework, quick fixes, workarounds, mistakes, delays, endless waiting, mis-scheduling, miscommunication, discarded materials, products allowed to expire, good products disposed of, food thrown away, supplies misused and discarded, missing keys, lost documents, equipment not ready when needed, out of date regulations, computer systems down, etc.

The good news is that an unsung benefit of systems thinking is that (1) it uncovers waste where others don't even notice it and (2) it knows how to deal with waste effectively and efficiently by redesigning processes and procedures to eliminate it.

In this chapter, we see personnel from the two healthcare systems trying to identify sources of waste in their hospitals and assess the damage it continues to do. They tell one story of squandering time, energy, effort, and prescription drugs in the pharmacy, and another about "potential waste" in failing to develop follow-up care plans for patients after they leave the hospital.

Later in the book you will feel the delight of these new systems thinkers as, again and again, they successfully find ways to reduce and eliminate waste in their units as they better serve patients.

WASTE IS NOT JUST ABOUT MONEY

Duplication, rework, lack of consistency, lack of supplies, waste of resources and money, and frustration permeate the entire hospital: the emergency room, the operating room, the nurses' station, the pharmacy, admission, billing, and purchasing. People involved at SSM Health Care and the Pittsburgh Regional Healthcare Initiative (PRHI) agree that there is huge waste, but offer different estimates of the percentage of waste going on in American hospitals.

> It is possible for our society to reduce the cost of health and medical care by 50 percent and simultaneously improve the outcomes for individual human beings.
>
> *Paul O'Neill, former U.S. Treasury Secretary,*
> *Former CEO, PRHI*

> It's not unrealistic at all to consider 40 percent and 50 percent waste in the healthcare system.
>
> *David Sharbaugh, Director of Quality Improvement,*
> *Shadyside Hospital, PRHI*

They all agree that waste is a major problem. More importantly, they identify different kinds of waste that many people might never label as waste.

Overuse of antibiotics in children for ear infections when none of them work anyway. Underused: Why don't more women get mammograms? And misuse. All of them, errors and waste. So, what I worry about today is that I think there's still at least 40 percent waste in the system.

Sister Mary Jean Ryan, FSM, RN, President & CEO,
SSM Health Care

All the patients who are not getting the flu shots or not getting proper immunizations or who are not having the proper screening test. That's a significant waste as well, because we are allowing people to get sick who could either be kept well or screened and their conditions identified earlier, so that we can treat them in a much less expensive way than we have to do after disease really manifests itself in a major way.

William P. Thompson, Senior Vice President,
Strategic Development, SSM Health Care

Forty percent waste in the system, and it is wasted time, it is wasted energy. It wastes peoples' creativity, their innovation. It wastes everything about the human person. That could possibly be the worst waste. People get so dragged down or pulled down into this. It's very demoralizing.

Sister Mary Jean Ryan, FSM, RN, President & CEO,
SSM Health Care

What we found was a lot of waste was not considered waste until we understood the process better.

Raymond LeBoeuf, CEO
PPG Industries

It used to be that these really expensive drugs applied to pretty uncommon diseases. Now what we're seeing are increasingly common diseases being treated with expensive drugs.

Donald J. Fetterolf, M.D.,
Chief Medical Officer, Highmark

The wasteful way that health care is delivered in just about every hospital in the country is well close to being insane.

Cliff Shannon, President, SMC Business Council,
Pittsburgh, PA

I don't think that we're wasteful as an industry. I think we're not as organized as we should be.

Kevin Kast, President,
SSM St. Joseph's Health Center

THE WASTE IN "WORK-AROUNDS"

Most experts have estimated that about one third of healthcare spending is wasted in one form or another. How does that happen? It's not because doctors and hospital administrators and nurses aren't trying to do the best they can. It's because the system itself is, at once, one layer of "work-arounds" and one layer of waste and mismanagement piled on another over a span of decades, until we have what Paul O'Neill has described as the world's largest remaining cottage industry delivering health care of the most sophisticated variety imaginable. There's bound to be waste, and that's what we need to reform.

Cliff Shannon, President, SMC Business Council,
Pittsburgh, PA

A "work-around" happens whenever a nurse or staff person needs something for a patient and it is not readily available—and should be! The nurse must work around the problem, perhaps by running from a patient's room to fetch something, making a phone call to track it down, finding something to substitute for it, and so on. The act of recognizing and compensating for an error-about-to-happen is also called a work-around.

Work-arounds abound in hospital work, and they are typically accepted as part of the job or business as usual. Identifying work-arounds as wasteful and frequently dangerous is a first step to eliminating them.

We in healthcare have devised unique work-arounds. For example, if a nurse goes to get a medication for a patient and the

28

medication isn't there, but she knows Mr. Smith in the next bed has that medication, she'll take it from Mr. Smith and give it to Mr. Jones, and then she'll go call the pharmacy and replace Mr. Smith's medication. We'll call that a work-around.

If you ask the nurse, "Is that a medication error?" she says. "Oh no, that's just part of doing my job." But it isn't. The medication should have been there at the right time for the right patient. It's what the nurses need to do their job. So many things happen in a hospital that are absolutely pitfalls for medication errors—serious medication errors—to occur. We learn to just work around them because we've gotten very good at it.

JoAnn V. Narduzzi, MD, Ph.D., VP of Academic Affairs,
Pittsburgh Mercy Health System, PRHI

Before, nurses would just go through the routine and if it was, for example, not getting a medication on time from pharmacy, they would be frustrated and they would continue to make their phone calls or follow whatever process it was to get that medication. But they would be frustrated...upset and...angry. But, most importantly, the patient wasn't getting what the patient needed.

Tina Danzuso, RN, Ward Director, General Surgery,
Shadyside Hospital, PRHI

That makes work harder to meet the patient's need. Providing the actual care isn't hard, it's the extra steps or non-value-added work that's out there.

Deborah Thompson, RN, Quality Trainer,
PRHI

If you can figure out a way to eliminate waste and eliminate the time that a nurse, for example, spends running around looking for things that they don't have, thereby making more of their time available to take care of the patients, then, yes, it could help because then you will have less of a need for additional nurses.

Connie Cibrone, President & CEO,
Allegheny General Hospital, PRHI

29

I learned through the Pittsburgh Regional Healthcare Initiative and through some of my observations that you'll see up to 40 to 50 percent of the work that people do is considered to be non-value added, meaning work that they're doing that does not support their day-to-day work. They might have to fetch a 2 by 2 gauze pad; they might have to search for a blood pressure cuff—things that should be right there waiting for them.

Deborah Ruckert, Quality Improvement Director,
Allegheny General Hospital, PRHI

As long as a defective or error-prone process remains in operation, nurses and other hospital personnel are forced to compensate for errors still happening.

For instance, let's suppose a physician writes an order and the pharmacist screens it. The pharmacist evaluates the order and puts a stop on it because it's the wrong dose, or there's a likely drug interaction, or it's the wrong drug, the wrong timing, or something else that could go wrong. That's what we call a pharmacy intervention of a physician order. In my hospital, depending upon the time of the year, we will have anywhere from 200 to 350 pharmacy interventions of physician orders on a monthly basis.

JoAnn V. Narduzzi, MD, Ph.D., VP of Academic Affairs,
Pittsburgh Mercy Health System, PRHI

WASTE IN THE PHARMACY

The pharmacy has its own special areas of waste, most of which are summed up in the word rework, doing things then doing them over again. The goal is to get it right the first time, every time, but often miscommunication rules. Kelley Wasicek, a Pittsburgh pharmacy manager, explains the view from the pharmacy.

Waste in pharmacy—defining waste as time, resources, money, frustration, and rework. You may find it unbelievable but it may be as much as 50 percent, the amount of time that we do things and then redo them. We waste people's time with unnecessary phone calls, chasing after information. We just can't always get it right the first time because the system is so complex. It's not a direct path from point A to point B. Fifty percent waste sounds outrageous but, upon closer inspection, I really don't think that's outrageous.

A strong concept in the Toyota production system principles is that you would hope not to pass the waste on to the next point in the system. So, a physician's poor handwriting may be the start of a waste process. If we're prescribing a medication that our patient needs for their care and the first step has a defect, then that's passed on. The waste is passed on because a phone call needs to be made, a physician needs to be contacted, interrupted, another order written, another order picked up, another medication prepared. So, illegible handwriting certainly contributes to the waste in the system. Physician order entry by computer is not the only answer. That will come with its own set of problems.

Rework and the waste come in many forms, whether it's people, time, resources—it could be anything. You send it out; it comes back. Why did we even send it out in the first place? So, if you get it right the first time, every time, there's no waste. Defect free.

For example, we would send a medication to a nurse in a vial, thinking it was ready to administer—nurse draws it up, goes into the patient's room, administers the med, and there we go. Little did we know that nurses didn't use this medication in a vial form every time we thought they did. Instead, they would draw the vial up, put it in a minibag and hang a drip. When we found this out, I said, "Well, if you're putting it in a bag, I can do that for you." So, in the course of 24 hours we made the change. We said, "Rather than send you medication in vial form, we'll send it with a bag attached, and there you are, it's ready to be administered." So we saved the nurse the time of going and finding a bag, a needle, a syringe, and tubing. We sent it to them in a much more ready to administer form. Had we not observed that work firsthand, we would still be sending stuff that they had to play with. So, it was in a matter of "you tell me what you want, and if I can do it, then certainly I'm glad

31

to do so." To be able to see other people's work and how you're connected to it is another tremendous benefit.

It's important to bring together all those involved in a wasteful process. For example, you might hand the physician the prescription he wrote, and say, "Hey, Doc. Here's why your patient didn't get that med within a reasonable amount of time." And he might say, "Oh! I wrote that." It's very interesting to see the light bulbs go off once you get the engagement of those that do the work.

Kelley A. Wasicek, R.Ph., Pharmacy Manager,
UPMC Presbyterian Hospital, PRHI

We have a physician who does a lot of wound care here. He writes a lot of wound-care orders, and some patients have lots of different wounds. So, when the orders go down to pharmacy, sometimes the staff doesn't know which wound he's talking about. His orders get very difficult to decipher. So, we came up with a special order sheet for this physician with all the different options for wound care. He just has to check it off. It really helps the pharmacist to decipher what's going on and what medications are needed.

Christine Quinn, Director of Professional Services,
LifeCare Hospitals of Pittsburgh, PRHI

We have Ph.D. pharmacists who man phone lines to intervene with physicians. This is a significant waste of time on the pharmacist's part. You're talking about a pharmacist having to get hold of 300 doctors a month. You know how difficult it is just to get hold of one. To get hold of three of them—up to 300 of them over a month's period of time—amounts to days and days of wasted pharmacy time, when those pharmacists could be interacting with patients, doing evaluations and histories, doing education, doing those kinds of things that enhance patient safety.

The other thing is it's also a waste of physicians' time because now they have to call back to the pharmacists to change their orders and rewrite orders. From that perspective alone it is a major issue. These are errors that don't reach the patient, so there's really no harm to the patient. The waste is the up-front cost in time for allied health professionals and for physicians.

JoAnn V. Narduzzi, MD, Ph.D., VP of Academic Affairs,
Pittsburgh Mercy Health System, PRHI

WASTE WHEN DISCHARGING PATIENTS

Before you get discharged from our hospital, we should be able to design the follow-up care for when you go home or wherever you go after the hospital. We should provide the infrastructure and the support such that you don't have to be readmitted on an unplanned basis. That's probably one of the most dramatic areas of waste—not being able to keep a patient well-managed and home, say, with congestive heart failure.

William Schoenhard, Executive VP & COO,
SSM Health Care

We've eliminated a lot of potential waste but I think that we've barely scratched the surface. I don't think that our services to-day are significantly better, but you know we may have ad-dressed only 5 percent to 10 percent of that waste. Whether you think it's 30 percent or 40 percent or 50 percent, there's still a tremendous amount that we can do to improve health care at a much lower cost and a much higher value than we are cur-rently providing.

William P. Thompson, Senior Vice President,
Strategic Development, SSM Health Care

Some Things to Remember From This Chapter

✓ Waste is a problem for all organizations, because it is hidden in many seemingly reasonable and traditional disguises.

✓ Waste is more and more difficult to identify as the organization becomes bigger and more complex.

✓ Waste can range from misuse of the time, talents and commitment of healthcare employees to poor inventory supply systems or failure to follow up with patients.

✓ Waste is not just money. The huge waste of effort and supplies in hospitals, if corrected, could reduce the cost of healthcare by as much as 50 per cent.

✓ One of the most useful powers of systems management is that it continually uncovers hidden waste and offers methods to reduce it.

CHAPTER 5

THE MOST DISABLING CHALLENGE WE FACED: REMOVING BLAME

Before we shifted to systems thinking, we were always looking for the bad apple. We believed that somewhere among the employees was a bad apple. If we could just get those employees out of here that weren't good employees this would be a great place. So, when we identified anybody likely to make a mistake or close to making a mistake, that was the person that we should fire. Often we did fire them, believing that by getting rid of them everything would get better. But what happened was that everything didn't get better.

Kevin Kast, President,
SSM St. Joseph's Health Center

THE BLAMING SICKNESS

We have all been told that money is the root of all evil. More recently, others have begun to suggest that *blaming* might be a better root for all evil. Blaming is a sickness that lies at the core of our culture. We learn its power as little children, seeing how frequently parents and older siblings use it to gain advantage or avoid punishment. It is pervasive in all aspects of life. From the Oval Office at the White House to the nursery schoolroom, when something goes wrong people's first reaction, even among children, is to look for someone to blame. Each one starts pointing the finger at someone else. President Harry S. Truman, expressing the accountability and responsibility of the highest U.S. office, once said, "The buck stops here." But evidently it doesn't stop there at all. Guilt can easily be reassigned to someone working on a lower rung of the totem pole.

But it is always some ONE!

Americans love to find someone—not themselves—to blame for anything that goes wrong. For big problems, we like to blame the government, the church, the community, the organization, the family, or a relationship. No matter. In an organization, we usually prefer to point the finger at some individual.

The media are obsessed with blame. When something bad happens, they get everyone to think in terms of blame, to ask, "Who is guilty?"

As we said in the Foreword, the modern world in its attachment to control and certainty looks for someone to blame when anything from natural disasters to epidemics occurs. In hindsight, someone should have warned or prevented whatever disaster. Scapegoating has biblical roots.

"Who is to blame?" Blaming is so omnipresent at home, at work, in school, in groups that we take its validity and usefulness for granted. It also proved to be a most disabling disease for the healthcare professionals we interviewed, and needed to be eradicated before they could begin healing their hospitals. How can mistakes in hospitals be removed if people hide them to avoid being blamed or punished?

Blaming leads to other unhelpful and sometimes destructive behavior. From fear of being blamed for some mishap and to save face, people involved will lie, point to someone else, hide the evidence, and distort the facts. They fear losing their jobs, being demoted, being treated as a "bad apple," being sued, and perhaps even being arrested.

Blaming never solved any problem or improved any process.

SYSTEMS THINKING AND BLAMING

One of philosopher W. Edwards Deming's 14 Points of quality management is to require all leaders, managers, and supervisors to *remove fear from the workplace.* Most workers fear being blamed when something goes wrong. Being blamed is especially feared among hospital workers, since a mistake, even a simple one, can sometimes prove deadly or costly.

Blame and fear are linked. Even the anticipation of being blamed generates fear. And when people are fearful and anxious in the workplace, their job does not receive their full attention and they cannot do their best work, especially the caring kind of tasks required in health care.

When people grow anxious or fearful, their nervous system automatically produces certain chemicals that prepare the body for fighting or fleeing, hardly the appropriate disposition for showing care and compassion.

Blaming others for mistakes that happen on the job is a major symptom of a fear-based working environment. Blaming generates feelings of opposition, secrecy, mistrust, and resentment, hardly the appropriate atmosphere for the intricate teamwork required to run a hospital.

An ambience of fear also stifles creativity. Someone who has fresh and helpful ideas to contribute will never mention them for fear of being laughed at or put down.

Fear curtails the continual improvement of processes and procedures, a key to successful systems management. Someone who sees a way to improve effectiveness or efficiency in a process will hold back for fear of triggering an angry reaction in a supervisor who may have instituted the process in its present form.

Fear also intensifies the ingrained American competitive attitude of win/lose. The blamer is always the winner. The one blamed is always the loser. Wholehearted teamwork is hardly possible when some on the team are one-up and others are one-down.

A healthcare organization cannot create win/win situations—where everyone comes out ahead—in an atmosphere of fear and blaming.

This chapter tells the story of how the people at PRHI and SSM Health Care realized what a deadly effect blaming had been having on their morale, and how this practice had been wielding its subtly corrosive power in their healthcare facilities.

What the staffs at PRHI and SSM Health Care discovered was that the system or a process within the system allowed the error or the problem. It could not be blamed on any particular individual. Experts estimate that some 90 percent of all defects in the delivery of a product or a service cannot be traced to an individual but come from the system. This is a difficult, counter-intuitive idea for Westerners. However it's a basic and important principle of systems thinking, a new mindset which has become increasingly necessary to effectively manage modern organizations. Once the hospital staff realized this, they made the

radical shift from finding someone to blame for every problem—eliminating the fear of being blamed—to redesigning the process where the
problem occurred so that it couldn't happen again.

> One thing we realized is that 99.9 percent of employees that
> come to work every day want to do a good job. They don't want
> to *not* do a good job. But whenever we had a problem or some-
> thing went wrong we asked the classic question: Whose fault
> is it? Whenever there was a failure, that was always our first
> question. We never questioned the process, that maybe there
> was something wrong in the way the process was designed.
>
> *Kevin Kast, President,*
> *SSM St. Joseph's Health Center*

BAD APPLES?

Once an organization begins to look at things from a systems perspective, it begins to move toward a blame-free culture. In this environment, people value learning from mistakes and fixing the process,
not replacing or blaming the people. One basic assumption of quality
management is that, for the most part, there are no bad apples; there
are no bad people, only bad processes, processes that need to be improved. Quality improvement requires a process-improvement focus.
Its aim is to make things better, to improve and facilitate interactions,
to reduce variation and improve outcomes.

A second assumption is that people learn something new only after
they recognize a mistake or a problem and devise a better way.

> The idea that desirable consequences and undesirable conse-
> quences in health care are due to good people or bad people is
> a faulty one. It's really an issue of good processes and bad pro-
> cesses. It's not a question of bad apples. It's rather a question of
> uncoordinated processes, fragmented processes or inefficient
> and ineffective processes. But changing processes is easier said
> than done. The effort is do-able, but it needs to involve all the
> stakeholders in the effort.
>
> *Alberto Colombi, MD, Chief Medical Officer,*
> *PPG Industries*

If you look at the literature on medical errors, much of it suggests that 80 to 85 percent of healthcare problems or errors occur because of defective processes or process issues. Research suggests that only 15 to 20 percent of errors may occur because of people problems or people issues.

Kevin Johnson, MD, VP for Medical Affairs,
SSM DePaul Health Center

People felt better if they had one person to blame. And they believed that if you could get rid of that person in some way shape or form then the hospital would be better off. What happens though is that people failed to recognize that if the problem was a process breakdown it doesn't matter who's going to make the same mistake the next time. The process will cause the same thing to happen. It's the definition of insanity to do the same thing over and over again expecting a different result.

Sister Mary Jean Ryan, FSM, RN, President & CEO,
SSM Health Care

In the past we have looked at an error as something that we had to blame somebody for. Now we have systems to look at, and instead we ask: "What's wrong with the way we do business that sets people up for medical errors?" For example, if we take a look at the major reason that we have medication administration errors, nurses will tell you it's because of the distractions and the pressures. We know that there is a nursing shortage, that our nurses are overworked and stressed, and the result of that is nursing error, and error results in medication errors.

JoAnn V. Narduzzi, MD, Ph.D., VP of Academic Affairs,
Pittsburgh Mercy Health System, PRHI

It's a completely different flip to shift from going for the bad apples to asking: Where are good people getting hurt? Where are they being caught up in bad processes and, in some cases, processes that don't work at all? That nurse who pulled a look-alike medication from the cart that was right next to the medication she meant to pull is not a bad apple. You can see that she's caught in a bad system in the way the drugs are stocked on that cart. And until we make that flip, away from looking for bad apples, we'll never be able to make improvements in the system. No matter how many good people we have, no matter how many motivational seminars we have, no matter how many employees we educate, if we can't fix the way medications are placed on that cart so that nobody can ever pull the wrong medication, that mistake will keep happening. We have to put processes in place for nurses so that, even under times of stress, those kinds of errors can't occur.

William Schoenhard, Executive VP & COO,
SSM Health Care

REPORTING ERRORS

As long as people fear that they will be blamed and held personally responsible for medical mistakes or pharmaceutical errors, they will avoid reporting them. As long as errors go unreported, faulty processes cannot be changed and improved. In other words, blame prevents errors, which are inevitable, from being corrected. So the errors and related unnecessary suffering and deaths continue.

It used to be a very big problem within the medical community to report errors because you were going to be punished, With PRHI, it's just the exact opposite. You are encouraged to report and there are no punitive repercussions from that at all. The whole goal is to get to the root of these problems so we can do away with them.

Ed Yonick, RN, Team Coordinator,
LifeCare Hospitals of Pittsburgh, PRHI

We have, I think, changed the conversation in the community around errors, and that has had a direct impact on how openly errors are discussed. Not completely open yet, not as much as we'd like, but more and more problems are being brought out into the open so they can be solved.

Kenneth Segel, former Executive Director
PRHI

We knew that the medication errors that were being reported were only the tip of the iceberg, that we were not really reporting all of them because it's a voluntary reporting system. Approximately two months after we initiated the hot line for reporting medical errors, the number of errors that were reported had tripled, and we have maintained this tripling rate on the hot line. I will tell you that even though we have tripled our hot line numbers, we still are not reporting them all.

JoAnn V. Narduzzi, MD, Ph.D., VP of Academic Affairs,
Pittsburgh Mercy Health System, PRHI

You know we've seen a tripling of the medication-error reporting rate across the community. We think that's good, but we realize that we have really 90-fold further to go. We still haven't brought anything near all of the errors out into the open so they can be solved.

Kenneth Segel, former Executive Director,
PRHI

The reporting of medication errors has increased to the extent now that people realize it's a much larger problem than anyone ever realized.

Marty Kurth, RN, Hospital Quality Trainer,

PRHI

For example, with the increased number of drugs the possibility of confusion around drug names or around drug uses increases exponentially, just because of the number of possible combinations.

We know mistakes and errors are going to occur. We just want to make sure that we learn from those mistakes so that, hopefully, no one will get harmed and, more importantly, that the same problem doesn't happen again.

Marty Kurth, RN, Hospital Quality Trainer,
PRHI

CREATING A BLAME-FREE ENVIRONMENT

The change starts in creating an environment where it's okay to make a mistake. We're very fortunate in our environment here at PRHI in that we've built, through the years, a culture of change, a culture of acceptance that says it's okay if you screwed up. The first time an employee approaches you and admits a mistake, the way you reply is most crucial. Suppose an employee comes to you, the supervisor, and says, "You know what? I hung that heparin wrong. I made a mistake. I think I may have overdosed that patient."

Your reaction as an individual is critical. If you say, "What in the heck did you do that for? How could you make such a mistake? What is wrong with you?" Versus. "I'm so thankful that you came forth and told me, because we need to do what's right for the patient. So let's get together and find out what we need to do and then let's find out why that happened."

Then, together you ask questions to get to the root of the problem. "Did you not have enough knowledge or training? Did the pump not work right? Did the pharmacy not get it mixed right? And let's fix things so we can prevent it for the next patient."

It's your response as a leader that creates the blame-free environment. It has to start with the CEO. And the VPs have to use the same kind of blame-free language. And the unit directors have to use the same words because, if at any point in that chain of command it's broken, it won't work because there will be some boss or supervisor that the average employee will say, "Well, I'm afraid if I tell her that I made that kind of mistake I'll get in trouble or I'll get fired."

It takes a lot of diligence and a lot of mutual support to create a blame-free atmosphere in a hospital. It's especially difficult when, as a leader, you hear about such crazy mistakes that you just want to pull your hair out and scream. At times like that, to stay calm and not overreact and to just really listen to what happened is a skill that takes time and reinforcement.

Tami Merryman, RN, Vice President, Patient Care Services,
Shadyside Hospital, PRHI

As long as people feel that they will be punished for things that they do, errors will go underground. Here, sometimes we're asked, "What is your error rate?" It's a rather peculiar question and sounds quite negative. However, we want more errors to be reported and more potential errors to be reported, because that's how we learn about flaws in our system and in our processes in order to fix them.

> *Grace Sotomayor, RN, Chief Nurse & VP Patient Services,*
> *SSM DePaul Health Center*

We have worked hard at changing the culture and allowing people to feel okay about reporting a problem or a mistake, so they can say, "I created a problem or I identified a problem, and I told other people about it. I didn't keep it to myself, even though I perhaps made a mistake, whether it was my fault or not."

The important thing is that it's okay to identify problems but it's really important that you tell everyone else that a problem occurred because, more than likely, others were involved in a similar problem in the past. And they were also afraid to tell anyone and admit to being involved in the mistake. If the workplace culture is non-punitive, employees see it as a safe environment for anyone to report problems and then, most importantly, they are willing to share that information so others can learn from it.

> *Marty Kurth, RN, Hospital Quality Trainer,*
> *PRHI*

When we begin to blame the process as opposed to the person, the person becomes much freer in sharing things that have gone wrong. That information is critical if we are to work to improve the process. I think that's part of the biggest issue.

> *William P. Thompson, Senior Vice President,*
> *Strategic Development, SSM Health Care*

NEAR MISSES

Besides identifying problems that have happened, people trained in quality improvement begin also to look for problems that "almost happened." This is a crucial step in error reduction and cannot be emphasized enough. Encouraging the reporting of near misses makes error proofing more robust and workers are more comfortable reporting near misses than actual errors. This provides more information to make process changes.

> In trying to come up with a revamped patient safety scheme, we started getting input from people who were closer to the bedside, people who were actually taking care of the patients, rather than managers who were sitting around talking about safety. So we developed a "near miss" form and it was really neat. With this emphasis we were hoping that people would tell us mistakes that "almost happened." Our task in the "near miss" form was to fix these things before they became problems. The first month I expected to get just a few reports back, and I got 20 near misses. The next month I got 30. It was exciting. We finally topped out at 50 a few months ago. It's been a very non-punitive experience. We had told people that they were not going to get in trouble for letting us know about these things, for pointing out shortcomings or things that we can do better.
>
> *Chris Grass, Clinical Pharmacist,*
> *SSM DePaul Health Center*

> We need to keep encouraging people to come forward with near misses, times when the patient isn't yet harmed. We've found we could often catch a mistake before the patient, say, got the wrong medication. We're trying to inculcate a culture where those near misses are brought to the surface so we can make the necessary process improvements that, next time, the near miss doesn't occur, and we avoid ending up with an actual injury to the patient.
>
> *William Schoenhard, Executive VP & COO,*
> *SSM Health Care*

Identifying near misses has been pretty wonderful for us. A lot of people are kind of scared of them, but we look at near misses as a chance to improve our safety in the hospital. Say, for instance, I go to a Pixus machine—that's where we get our medication. I go in there and I'm supposed to pull out Valium. If maybe there's something that only looks like a Valium tablet or it's the wrong dosage of Valium, what I'll do is call the pharmacy and tell her that there's a medicine in this Pixus that shouldn't have been in here. It was placed on the wrong number. She'll come down. She'll look at the Pixus. She'll get it straight.

We have a form for near misses. If you fill it out, they give you movie tickets or some reward just for identifying something that could have been a mistake.

Anita Montgomery, RN, ER Team Coordinator,
SSM DePaul Health Center

One of our goals in the medication error reduction team has been to increase the number of near misses or errors that never reach the patient by a significant number, by 50 percent. We have been able to achieve that. And the way we have done that is by actually rewarding people who tell us about things that they've found and that they've fixed.

It's important that employees who work within any industry feel no fear about speaking up when they identify something inappropriate happening or about to happen. For example, whether you look at the Challenger disaster or whether you look at the Enron scandal, or whether you look at the scandals in healthcare that are in the public news everyday, they would probably not have occurred had employees working in those industries felt able to say, "Stop the presses. We should not be doing this. This is inappropriate. It's against our values."

At SSM Health Care, the more that we can empower our staff to say, "This is not right, we need to fix this," and we stop errors from reaching the patient, this will help solve some of the issues in health care.

Grace Sotomayor, RN, Chief Nurse & VP Patient Services,
SSM DePaul Health Center

Within our system we try to look at the process level so we can espouse a blame-free culture. We separate learning from mistakes, and fixing the process not replacing the people. So much of basic CQI is that there are no bad apples, there are no bad people. Its bad processes. And so how can we have a process focus to make things better? More systematically we learned to reduce variation and improve outcome.

Paula Friedman, Vice President, Systems Improvement,
SSM Health Care

People don't want to make mistakes, but sometimes processes that are in place can cause mistakes because of breakdowns from one department to another and so we focus on the process we need to improve, not on the individual.

Maggie Fowler, Vice President of Patient Services,
SSM St. Joseph's Health Center

New ways to see and think about blame were just the beginning of the unexpected changes required to begin to heal hospitals. In the next chapter, healthcare professionals tell how they begin to view the entire hospital in a wider, more effective way and imagine startling new improvements.

SOME THINGS TO REMEMBER FROM THIS CHAPTER

✔ Blaming an individual is the direct opposite of systems thinking; it is unproductive and raises fear.

✔ Blame says the outcome is due to the individual rather than a result of the system.

✔ In systems thinking there are no bad people, only bad processes that need to be improved.

✔ Blame, a radical form of waste, creates fear, stops creativity and causes people to hide mistakes.

✔ A culture of blame will ruin any attempt at healing the organization.

PART II:

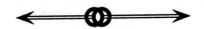

Solutions

CHAPTER 6

SYSTEMS THINKING AND CONTINUAL PROCESS IMPROVEMENT

This is not about the people who work in hospitals. This is about the fact the processes in hospitals are so broken that there really isn't any way for people whose good intentions are clear to impact the system positively without really going through the stages of process improvement.

Sister Mary Jean Ryan, FSM, RN, President & CEO, SSM Health Care

SYSTEMS AND PROCESSES AND THE DELIVERY OF CARE

The most important thing the executives at SSM Health Care and PRHI learned was that any hospital or large organization is a single system. To change and improve such a complex system, the people in an organization need to learn a revolutionary new mindset that gives them new eyes and a new understanding of their work, their customers, and their fellow workers.

This mindset is called systems thinking. It is a mindset that needs to be learned consciously. In our task-oriented society, we tend to be habitual, unconscious, single-event thinkers. Such a mindset may have sufficed in managing the details of a hospital in an earlier, simpler time. But it is sorely inadequate in today's complex and constantly changing culture.

A healing transformation happened in these institutions—not because employees learned some new methods or practices or because everyone started working harder—but because the employees learned to think in a new way.

This new way of thinking gave them new eyes to see things they had never noticed before. With this new thinking, they could also recognize ways to make improvements they never imagined before. Suddenly, they could identify interconnections between people and tasks they had not noticed. Systems thinking gave them an expanded perspective for looking at processes and procedures they had been performing for years. It allowed them to create new ways to make their work more efficient and effective—again and again. They learned to grasp entire processes and whole systems, instead of just lists of department responsibilities and job descriptions. They learned to observe not only the obvious actions of people but also the more subtle and intangible interactions that occurred among them—and that made all the difference.

The systems thinking mindset is the primary source of the healing transformation in these healthcare organizations. Do not be distracted by new methods or techniques for improvement—like using flow charts or the PDSA cycle. To use these tools effectively requires systems thinking and "new eyes" to see what needs to be improved and how best to make that improvement.

Later in this chapter, you will hear how the staff at PRHI used this new way of thinking to develop *learning lines*. Here, using a small part of the unit as a laboratory, the staff can formulate and test ideas for possible improvements, then continually refine those improvements until they can be applied throughout the entire unit.

We also tell the story of how in an SSM facility doctors and nurses used systems thinking to manage the blood sugar levels of critically ill patients, thereby saving many lives and much money.

Finally, we close the chapter with a fascinating story of how an SSM hospital used systems thinking and its mandate for continual improvement to revolutionize services in an emergency room, so that today more than 90 percent of the patients who come to the emergency room without a life-threatening accident or illness are under active care within 30 minutes. Those with life-threatening problems are under active care within 30 seconds.

SYSTEMS THINKING

Few people truly understand the mindset called systems thinking and how different it is from single-event thinking. People commonly assume that a system—a hospital, for example—is the sum of its parts;

that is, each one doing his or her job, giving their best efforts with enthusiasm and commitment will create excellent health care. Managers who make that assumption are not systems thinkers but single-event thinkers. Such thinking, even with dedicated employees, has led many an organization, including hospitals, down a path into inefficiency and ineffectiveness. An effective system will naturally be more than the sum of its parts because of the quality of the *interactions* of the people with each other and the machines they use. Systems thinkers quickly become aware of how their work fits into the system—e.g., the hospital—and the processes, which make up the system.

Eunice Halverson, Corporate Vice President of SSM Health Care's Quality Resource Center, explains this big difference, when she talks about a process, which is simply systems language to describe a group of people working together to produce a service or product for a customer.

> When you look at a process you can actually look at the steps of the process that make up the whole. For some reason, if we are task oriented or single-event thinkers, our brains don't see that way, don't work that way. It's like we are each working in a silo. I'm going to do this task while others might be doing a couple of other tasks at the same time. But we don't seem to see them as tasks that integrate with one another, that interface.
>
> *Eunice Halverson, Corporate Vice President,*
> *Quality Resource Center, SSM Health Care*

On the contrary, a systems thinker sees an organization such as a hospital, not as the sum of its parts but primarily as the *product of its interactions*. A system is not measured merely by what people are *doing individually* but how well they are *working together*—interacting and interfacing. It is the quality of their interactions that makes an organization greater—or lesser—than the sum of its parts.

A good example of a system is the human body. It is not just the sum or accumulation of its parts, because the whole body is greater than the sum of its parts. What makes the whole greater are the *interactions* of the parts.. For example, your hand alone does not write a letter, slice a tomato, brush your teeth, work the TV remote or turn the steering wheel of your car. Every one of those activities requires the interaction and precise coordination of fingers, wrists, arms, shoulders, spine, and eyes, plus a lot of simultaneous neuronal firing in the brain stem, limbic system, and the cortex. It is your whole body—the system—that writes, slices, brushes, pushes and turns.

In any organization as in any organism, there are many more inter-actions than actions. While actions are usually quite visible and mea-surable, interactions are, for the most part, intangible and invisible. Interactions happen in a realm of "between"—in that intangible space between the parts or people. Thus, as a whole, a system is for the most part something invisible and intangible. In fact, it is important to remember that what really makes a system powerful and gives it wholeness is mostly invisible.

A Shared Aim Unifies and Integrates

What makes a system a system and gets all of its parts interacting efficiently and effectively is that the parts have a _shared aim_. For ex-ample, the shared aim of all your bodily parts is to keep you healthy and alive. Unless everyone in a complex social system, like a hospital, agrees and commits to a shared aim, there cannot be a system. They are merely a group of people working side by side with many differ-ent aims or purposes.

It is also true that each employee or member of a system may have his or her own personal agenda for working in this organization. So, if a system is to be greater than the sum of its parts, its shared aim needs to be so desirable, powerful, stimulating, and inspiring that it embraces and helps fulfill each one's personal agenda. For a hospital, the only possible unifying aim is to totally focus on the health and care of the patient.

Therefore, the first order of business in creating a successful complex social system is to find a powerfully inspiring aim to which everyone is ready and willing to commit. Once this shared aim is clear to everyone, then, and only then, may the processes or tasks of various teams be studied and redesigned to improve the interaction of people and the flow of work. The criterion of improvement is: Does this change further the organization's shared aim or not? In the case of hospitals, the cri-terion might be: Does this change in a process promote perfect patient care, or not? Though the aim is perfect patient care, leaders know that the benefit of using systems thinking to achieve this will also include increased satisfaction for hospital staff and reduction in costs.

SYSTEMS, SUBSYSTEMS, AND PROCESSES

Like any large complex social or manufacturing organization, a hospital as a healthcare system is made up of many subsystems, and each of those subsystems is made up of many processes. The easiest mistake to make is to think of any of those hospital subsystems or processes as independent of any other in the whole system.

According to Raymond LeBoeuf, CEO of PPG Industries in Pittsburgh and strong supporter of the Pittsburgh Regional Healthcare Initiative,

> Process improvement is key to health care just as it is key to all business success. Everybody involved in the process must, first of all, know there's a process. That sounds simple but I think a lot of times people think that they're a part of a group of individual contributors that act independently of one another. But that isn't the case. There is connectivity in what's being done, and in hospitals and in medicine, that connectivity must be strong. There is a mosaic in medical care that needs to be understood by all of those involved. They must understand what each person's role is, not only their own, and what everybody else is depending on throughout the value chain here in hospital care.

Paula Friedman, a systems improvement vice president at SSM Health Care, adds,

> So much of health care has been task oriented. It's fixing this issue or that issue. Being task oriented doesn't understand the context of the whole patient view—the patient perspective—how what we do impacts patients personally, their families, and their lives. It's that compassionate difference in how we deliver that care as well as the tactical things that we do each day.

Only when patient care and safety are uppermost in the minds of the hospital staff can they predict whether a proposed change or redesign in a subsystem or process will be an improvement. People at SSM Health Care and PRHI, committed to continual improvement of their processes, learned always first to ask themselves, "Will this change help improve patient care and safety? Will it free up doctors, nurses and other healthcare personnel to spend more time caring for patients?" For each of the two hospital systems, this perspective, above all, has been the core of their successful transformation.

The leaders began to understand that their healthcare institutions had become sick because they had lost sight of their true purpose, the care and safety of patients. The problem wasn't the people who worked in hospitals. The problem was the system, its lack of a shared focus and its defective processes. Here is the story in their own words.

> Many things you do because that's the way you've always done them. So, we took our blinders off and said, "That may be the way we've always done it, but how do we shorten these steps? How do we get from here to where we want to be?" For example, how do we find a bed for a patient quickly? By doing that, we changed our process.
>
> *Maggie Fowler, Vice President of Patient Services,*
> *SSM St. Joseph's Health Center*

> We were like a lot of organizations that in trying to fix a problem we added staff. That was always the first thing we came up with. We said, "We could move this process along if we just added another nurse over here, or we just added another technician over here, or if we just put another room over here." What we learned when we spent that year developing quality systems is that our processes were flawed. The last thing we do now when we want to solve a problem is to add people. The last thing we do is add resources. Instead, we look at our design and we improve our design.
>
> *Kevin Kast, President,*
> *SSM St. Joseph's Health Center*

> So much of organizational policy is doing things because that's the way we've always done them. Now, we really assess why we do the things that we do. Everything that we do now, I would say, is more intentional than ever before. We understand the questions—Whom do we serve? What do they want

55

from us? How do we know?—and we put that into place with defined measurements. So, it's not just delivering exceptional health care but understanding how we define it and what that means.

Paula Friedman, Vice President, Systems Improvement,
SSM Health Care

What we've accomplished over the last 13 years is to have people truly recognize that the delivery of care is a process. It may not be as rigid as building an automobile but it is still a process. Now we collect information on everybody that comes through our front door or through our ER. We analyze that information. We take that analysis and draw some conclusions from it; based upon those conclusions we design a treatment plan. We treat the patient according to that plan.

We evaluate the results. If the results have achieved the objectives we have established, then the patient is usually discharged to another level of care. If not, we go back and reassess it. That's basically the Plan-Do-Check-Act cycle we follow.

William P. Thompson, Senior Vice President,
Strategic Development, SSM Health Care

One of the hallmark methods for quality improvement is called PDSA (Plan-Do-Study-Act) or, as Thompson called it, PDCA, that is Plan-Do-Check-Act. Before a process change is implemented throughout an organization, it is tested by a PDCA cycle. The test begins with a well laid-out Plan, which is then tried or tested on a small scale (Do). The results of the test are then Studied or Checked, and perhaps modified. Finally, the newly or re-designed process is put into place in the system (Act). The PDSA cycle may be repeated again and again, since every process is always open to continual improvement.

We believe that all work is part of a process and because of that we can improve it. And we believe that people are not the cause of the issues but rather broken processes that we need to fix.

Eunice Halverson, Corporate Vice President,
Quality Resource Center, SSM Health Care

There is not one hospital across the country that doesn't have a process they can improve.

Brenda Peterson, RN, Patient Access Director,
SSM St. Joseph's Health Center

And so all of the work that we do in caring for the patient is a process. (That's how it is in manufacturing also.) So, if we look at that process and flowchart the steps in the process, then we can find ways to reduce the time. We can eliminate the waste, and we can get better care to the patient by making it a better process.

Eunice Halverson, Corporate Vice President,
Quality Resource Center, SSM Health Care

A flowchart is a sketch or map of a process or a system that graphically describes the flow of activity from beginning to end. Each step in the process is boxed and labeled, and arrows indicate the direction of the flow of activity from one box to another. Some flowcharts are rather simple because the process they describe is merely a series of consecutive steps, one following the other, from beginning to end. Most processes, however, are quite complicated, involving branching arrows and feedback loops, so their flowcharts reflect their complexity. Creating flowcharts is an often-used skill learned by every systems thinker.

For example, in the work of the pharmacy one apparently simple process that could be flowcharted is receiving a doctor-written prescription, reading it, and filling it. From start to finish, its flowchart sounds like an easy three-step process. The pharmacy team may at first draw it on a chalkboard in this elementary form:.

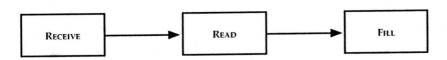

However, any pharmacist will point out that there are many missing steps in this flowchart. For instance, during the reading step what if the doctor's handwriting is unclear? What if two drugs have almost the same spelling and you're not sure which one the doctor wants?

Or what if you're not sure whether the doctor wrote a six or a zero in one place? Or what if a decimal point is unclear, and you're not sure whether the doctor wanted the dosage to be 1.0 cc. or 10 cc?

So that the pharmacist may catch any near misses when written information is unclear, the team may have to add branching steps to their flowchart, such as telephoning the doctor, clarifying the drug or dosage, and amending the prescription.

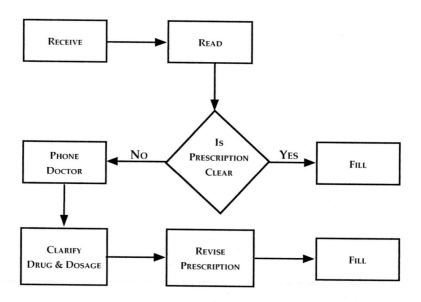

Again, in the Fill step, the pharmacist points out there are other considerations. For instance, it is essential to verify the identity of the patient who is to receive the medication, since often there may be another patient with the same name in a large hospital. Therefore, a process for verifying the patient must be put into the flowchart. Also, if this is a new drug for this patient, or a new doctor prescribing a medication, the drug must be checked for possible interactions with other drugs the patient is currently taking. If another question arises, perhaps more phone calls to doctors may be required, which will require another branching process in the flowchart. And so on.

Eventually, a more complete flowchart is drawn that fills in the missing steps, is designed to catch any mistakes, ensures that the shelf supply of the drug is not running low, ensures security and safety for any dangerous drugs, and provides the drug in proper form (vial, tablet, liquid, syringe, etc.) In many cases, processes like filling a prescription that appear simple at first may ultimately require dozens of steps and go off into many branches before the process is actually completed and the medication is delivered to a patient properly and safely.

JUST TWO MORE DEFINITIONS

In this book, you are going to come across two words that are quite common in every day conversation, "system" and "complex." These words are used in a special, technical sense.

Whenever the word "system" appears, it refers to an interacting arrangement of things, ideas or people that forms not only a simple union or unity, but also an interacting whole that can be greater than the sum of all its parts.

The word "complex" is almost always used as an adjective to identify a certain kind of system. A "complex system" refers to a special category of systems, namely, a system of interacting relationships involving things, ideas and people _that is constantly changing or re-adapting itself in response to internal as well as external forces._

An ocean, a human body and the weather are examples of complex systems that are constantly changing or re-adapting themselves in response to both internal and external forces. A hospital is, of course, another example of a complex system.

A complex system must never be mistaken for a _complicated system._ The words "complex" and "complicated" have significantly different meanings in systems language.

A "complicated system" consists of an intricate combination of interacting parts whose components work in a predictably fixed pattern. An auto, a computer and a camera, are examples of complicated systems. Once you have designed and built an auto, computer or camera, you can assemble the same set of parts over and over again and, predictably, get the same working results. Most importantly, none of these complicated systems keeps adapting and re-inventing or changing itself as it functions. Consistently predictable behavior of a complicated system, like a computer or a camera, is one of the things you are paying for when you buy it. Such systems, though intricate and complicated, should be dependably repetitive in how they work.

ADD A HUMAN BEING

However, in most cases, when you add a user to any complicated system like an auto, computer or camera it becomes a complex system. Once you add people to almost any mechanical or electronic system, it becomes complex, precisely because humans have free will and in their interaction with that auto, camera or computer may begin adapting and changing the ways they use it.

As highly complex systems, hospitals involve hundreds of people with free will using hundreds of pieces of complicated machinery and equipment and following hundreds of processes. You can imagine what may happen when each of these people begins adapting and changing the way they use equipment and the ways they interact with each other.

Complex systems such as the ocean, the human body and the weather are still so incompletely understood that we may never feel capable of understanding or dealing with many of the behaviors and/or changes they manifest. The forces and/or components that make up an ocean, the human body or the weather produce a system of interactive relationships that are continuously in a state of change—some easily observed, some not. If the changes are slight, there are usually no major problems to deal with. However, when larger and more complex systems, like hospitals or oceans or weather patterns, are not sufficiently understood, the results they produce, even ones that are unintended, can be devastating.

CONSTANT AWARENESS

When attempting to manage a complex system like a hospital, any management approach will usually work for at least a while, but only for a while. This is inevitable because the interacting parts and relationships that make up that system are always in a process of adapting to new forces—new equipment, new regulations, new employees, new diseases, new costs, new expenses, etc.—that result in new problems, bottlenecks, conflicts and confusion requiring a new management approach. Complex system problems can only be solved for a while. And only then by a constant awareness and analysis of the changes that have produced the newest problem needing a new resolution.

National health care is an immensely complex system. Within that system each of the more than 6,000 hospitals in this country forms its own local complex system. To solve the problems of those local complex systems, people in them must be adaptable and willing to change—continually! Since people do not like to change—no matter what they say—getting them to change continually will never be easy. However, when the personnel in the hospitals we studied learned the new mindset called systems thinking, they not only found it easy to change continually, they also discovered the joy of doing it. They saw that by continually adapting the ways they worked together they improved their ability to care for their patients and, at the same time, made their own work easier and more satisfying.

In the next chapter, hospital staffs explain how they successfully practiced systems thinking.

Some Things to Remember From This Chapter

✓ Any hospital or large organization is a single system.

✓ To improve this changing, complex social system, the people in it need to learn and practice systems thinking

✓ Systems thinking, remember, teaches people to recognize problems and to design improvements.

✓ It is a new mindset that gives people a new understanding of connections, work, customers and fellow workers.

✓ This mindset must be consciously learned, because most people are habitual and unconscious non-systems or single-event thinkers.

✓ In systems thinking, looking for improvement never ends.

CHAPTER 7

SYSTEMS THINKING IN ACTION

*When we first started, we all thought we had problems
but we had no idea of the extent of the problems. Now
that we have a database where we're actually measuring and collating what we do, we are really beginning
to understand that we have processes in our hospitals
that for the most part set up our clinicians in an atmosphere that allows them to make errors. Before now, we
used to look at our patients as a one-on-one individual
encounter, and we did not look at the processes of care
within our institutions. And if you look at why we
create errors, it's because the processes that we have in
place either stress our nurses or don't allow physician
interactions correctly. The problems that we have are
not mostly people but more the system.*

JoAnn V. Narduzzi, MD, VP. Academic Affairs,
Pittsburgh Mercy Health System, PRHI

A SYSTEMS THINKING "LEARNING LINE" AT PRHI

At PRHI, they work with a concept called a *learning line*. The *line*
refers to a slice of an organizational system, which is, typically, a process the hospital uses. The *learning* part means that the line, or process, is seen as a laboratory where people can make experiments. It
is a metaphor adapted from employees using continual improvement
techniques in an automotive production line and used by hospital employees in viewing and improving various processes in a hospital. For
example, one learning line might identify a problem in an inpatient
unit on Four West. Using the *learning line* strategy, the staff there can
formulate and test hypotheses about possible improvements by actually implementing and refining them until the improvements become
stable in that unit.

In the flush of excitement at their success, it's tempting for people
on Four West to rush off and want to apply this improved process on
every other inpatient unit in the hospital, saying, "We've solved this

problem on Four West. Can't we take it to the intensive care unit and deploy it there, too, right away?"

Copying other people's successes does not work in systems theory. A change in process must be tested and re-invented for each new site. Front line workers become believers when they see how much better a process they developed works instead of an edict or change ordered by higher management.

Peter Perreiah, PRHI's director, cautions:

> We encourage people to come to our unit and look at the counter measures and see if what we did might actually solve problems they're encountering. We encourage them not to stop there. We want them to actually talk to the people on Four West who use the new system, so they begin to understand the ins and outs, the pitfalls of running that system, what Four West experienced in developing that system. Then, we encourage them to examine their own system and understand their own current condition. Often, the motivation or the counter measure needed to solve their problem is not the same, because it's occurring under different circumstances, and it would be inappropriate to implement it under those different circumstances.

UNDERSTANDING PROCESSES

> Processes are easier to fix than people. A person comes to us with a certain set of skills and we have to recognize the talents they bring to the job, but we also have to ask them to help us design a process that allows them to do the best job they can. And so by focusing on the process and looking for ways to change that process to deliver better care, more cost-effective care, truly frees up the individual because it takes the onus off the individual and allows them to apply their talents, skills, and creativity in a much different fashion.
>
> _William P. Thompson, Senior Vice President,_
> _Strategic Development, SSM Health Care_

We use flowcharts a lot to visualize. We use them often when discussing our policies and procedures because you can actually see the flow from start to finish. That really helps people to understand how the process works and how it can be improved. And this gets us back into that mindset that's always making improvements.

Eunice Halverson, Corporate Vice President,
Quality Resource Center, SSM Health Care

We have never observed and prepared the healthcare team in the same way the airlines would a cockpit crew or the in-flight team around an airplane that is about to take off. Preparing healthcare teams has really been treated rather casually.

Karen Wolk Feinstein, Chair & Founder of PRHI,
President Jewish Healthcare Roundtable

What we found was that a lot of waste was not considered waste until we understood the process better. What was once valuable input and necessary steps in the process became waste, once we understood how the process could be better run. And that improving of the process is continual. I think that's an aspect of quality management that one has to recognize. There's no absolute here. Every process is continually reviewed, it is continually improved.

Raymond LeBoeuf, CEO
PPG Industries

SSM HEALTH CARE AND CQI

For the people at SSM Health Care, their inclusive term for systems thinking, systems management, and process improvement is CQI, which stands for Continual Quality Improvement. CQI represents a systems-thinking mindset as well as a management approach and various methods and techniques used to transform a healthcare system.

In May of 1990,...we rolled out our CQI journey. We were going to adopt the principles of continual quality improvement, the purpose of which was to change the culture of this organization. It was not necessary to get better, but to create a culture committed to getting better, which we thought was really the foundation of what we do.

> *William P. Thompson, Senior Vice President,*
> *Strategic Development, SSM Health Care*

We're trying to inculcate a culture where near misses are sur-faced. Then we can make the process improvement so that the near miss doesn't occur again and we end up with an actual injury to the patient.

> *William Schoenhard, Executive VP & COO,*
> *SSM Health Care*

SSM Health Care CEO, Sister Mary Jean Ryan, formulates the es-sence of CQI in a sentence: "How do you say in a sound bite what CQI is? I look on it as a way of thinking and behaving that utilizes people's talents and skills in teams to improve care for the people that we serve."

At DePaul Health Center we review each thing we do and look for opportunities to do it better. Even when there's not an error or a mistake or something bad happening, we take input from everybody and try to do it better each time. From the first day in orientation, we talk about continuous quality improvement. It's not just a slogan. CQI is how we do what we do each day.

> *Russ Schroeder, CTC Telemetry Division,*
> *SSM DePaul Health Center*

CQI is a framework for decision-making. What it does as far as strategic planning goes is help us identify who our customers are, what is happening in our market, what our growth poten-tial is. What are the things that we're doing well? What are the things we need to do better? What are the things we shouldn't do any more because the market has changed? It also helps us identify where we should invest our capital dollars for the fu-ture.

Our focus is on: What do we need to continuously improve? Even though we began this CQI initiative quite a few years ago, we still meet every two weeks to ask ourselves, "What are the barriers to success? What are the issues we're dealing with now?" And we focus on what the issues are, not necessarily on how well individuals are doing.

Maggie Fowler, Vice President of Patient Services,
SSM St. Joseph's Health Center

Constantly finding ways to do better, to improve upon the ways that you've been doing it. If you have a better way, you don't resort to old ways. You continually try your best to make things better.

Matt Clausen, Dietary Supervisor,
SSM St. Joseph's Hospital West

If we find out that another hospital is performing better in how they manage heart attacks, we can go to that hospital and ask them, "What are you doing differently?" And then we can re-analyze what we're doing ourselves. We can use some of the information or observe some of the best practices that they use there, and adapt them in our own hospital to do a better job ourselves.

Kevin Johnson, MD, VP for Medical Affairs,
SSM DePaul Health Center

Any time we see something that could be a problem or might cause the patient problem, we fill out this simple form. The CQI team then reviews it, where everyone gives input. All staff are asked to give input to help figure out a better way to do this process and thus have a better result for our patients.

Patricia Abramczyk, RN, Staff Nurse, Orthopedics,
SSM DePaul Health Center

Over the last two years we have dramatically improved our performance. An example of that would be: Can you document giving aspirin in the emergency room for an acute myocardial infarction? And we were probably 40 to 50 percent compliant in that. And now we're 95 to 98 percent compliant.

Kevin Johnson, MD, VP for Medical Affairs,
SSM DePaul Health Center

A CASE STUDY:
MANAGING BLOOD SUGAR LEVELS OF CRITICALLY ILL PATIENTS

Our goal is to continually improve the quality of the care we deliver to patients in the intensive care unit and, in my role as vice president of clinical affairs, to extend that quality improvement to patients throughout the hospital regardless of their disease.

Our most recent and compelling case for improvement has been in the management of blood sugar in critically ill patients. We came across some information from Europe, where surgical critical care patients who had blood sugars managed to normal had about a 40 percent reduction in their hospital mortality—regardless of whether or not they were diabetic, regardless of what their underlying disease was. So we went through a stepwise process to reduce our blood sugar targets from about 175—which is where we were two years ago—to the current target of 120. And in the last 20 months we've seen our intensive care unit mortality drop from about 5.5 percent to about 3.2 percent.

The article about this was already published in the *New England Journal of Medicine,* not by me, but by Dr. Vandenberg. That's where I found the original article, in the November 2001 issue. The interesting thing is Vandenberg set a target of 108 as an optimal blood sugar level. That's where he ended up. I don't think you need to get quite that low to see the benefits that he has shown, which is why we gradually reduced our blood sugars in a stepwise fashion. We found that once our blood sugars were (reliably) under about 140, we saw a dramatic reduction in mortality that's persisted.

Every time our blood sugars rise up much above that value, we seem to lose the benefit. As a matter of fact, we in medicine have known for at least 25 years that high blood sugar reduces the ability of the white cells to deal with infection.

Clearly SSM's philosophy of continual quality improvement makes the implementation of this kind of a program much easier. We're blessed at this hospital with a nursing staff that shows very little turnover, so we have a lot of continuity with our nurses and a lot of buy-in to new programs. This was a program that had almost immediate nursing buy-in. In fact, they wanted the program to go faster, once we got started.

We have reduced the whole hospital's average blood sugar from about 165 to 135. That's every patient throughout the hospital, and that's a dramatic reduction. We've reduced the number of acute and in-hospital diabetic complications from about 13.5 percent to about 5 percent.

Filippo Ferrigni, MD, VP, Critical Care Director,
SSM St. Joseph's Health Center

Continual Quality Improvement also led to one of SSM's greatest accomplishments—taking Dr. Ferrigni's pioneering work at one hospital and implementing these changes at all SSM's ICUs in four states.

A Case Study:
SSM Health Care Emergency Room Story

When you ask people on the street what their biggest complaint is about hospital emergency rooms, the answer is universally the same: the seemingly endless waiting to be seen by a medical professional.

Through focus group interviews with patients we realized that one of the number one things that patients were interested in was timely health care in the emergency department. They anticipated two- to four-hour waits in emergency departments and that was one of their number one concerns.

Tim Thompson, DO, Emergency Room Director,
SSM St Joseph's Hospital West

Most communities have a love/hate relationship with emergency departments. They either love them to death because something tragic happened and we saved their loved one, or their experience has only been ugly and they've had to wait too long and nobody talked to them, and the nurse was rude, and, you know, on and on and on and on.

Kristine Mims, Clinical Director Emergency Department,
SSM St. Joseph's Health Center

When we started thinking about it, we were causing frustration and anger in 60,000 or 75,000 people a year, not counting
the additional people that came in with them when they came
to the hospital.

Kevin Kast, President,
SSM St. Joseph's Health Center

This is a McDonald's kind of drive-through world and patients
want to come to the emergency room and watch their watches
and be in and out because they have to move on to their next
thing to do for the day. So, waiting creates a lot of unhappi-
ness with the patient population that comes to the emergency
room.

Kristine Mims, Clinical Director, Emergency Department,
SSM St. Joseph's Health Center

We found a hospital in Detroit that had a program that they
refer to as their 30/30 Program. The idea is in 30 seconds they
will make certain that anyone that comes into the hospital with
life or limb-threatening chest pain, whatever, they will be seen
immediately. But all others would be under active care within
30 minutes. We wanted to replicate that program in our hospital. In the process of replicating that program we found out it's
not just the ER that has to reorganize, redevelop, and redesign
processes, you have to do this throughout the hospital.

Kevin Kast, President,
SSM St. Joseph's Health Center

The 30/30 Program appealed to the SSM administration, and they
wanted to try it. Even though they had had successes using the CQI
principles for a number of years, they felt that the solution would be a
quick and simple one. They were wrong. But they were committed.

We just felt that if the doctors would work harder and the nurses
would work harder we could get people through. And then we
found out that this was going to require a systemic change in
our whole organization and a totally different culture. So, it
took us at least a year to organize the hospital and get all of our

employees committed to this, that the 30/30 program was part of their job, even though they didn't work in the emergency services department.

Kevin Kast, President,
SSM St. Joseph's Health Center

If you try and do it just in the emergency department, it will fail. You have to have the support of housekeeping to get the room clean so you can get the patient out of the bed here in the ER and into the hospital. You have to have the commitment of administration to allow you to add resources if you find you need resources. You have to have the commitment of the kitchen. Everyone, nursing up on the floors. It has to be a whole institution-wide initiative.

Tim Thompson, DO, Emergency Room Director,
SSM St Joseph's Hospital West

And so every department identified what their role was going to be in the initiative, what they would do to help support it. And then we tested it, and we measured it, and we continue to measure every single day to make sure everyone is doing what he or she said they were doing.

It's like a fine-tuned machine. You need to make sure in an engine that all the different parts are working together to help that car or that engine run smoothly. And this is very similar. In order to achieve the outcomes we want in getting the patient into the hospital and making their experience in the emergency department a positive one, it takes everyone in the building to make it successful.

Maggie Fowler, Vice President of Patient Services,
SSM St. Joseph's Health Center

Many of the staff resisted. They said, "How can we work harder when we're already working as fast as we can? If we try to get people through faster, we'll make mistakes and we won't do things right. We're too busy and overloaded already."

We certainly got some push-back from our employees, you know. "It's more work. Why do we want to work harder? We're not going to be able to do it. We're not going to be successful. This is too big of an expectation. If it was easy to do, why aren't other hospitals doing it?"

Kevin Kast, President,
SSM St. Joseph's Health Center

We said, "We're too busy. We've got too many ambulances. We have too many things to do. There's no way we can do this." However, in really looking at it and everybody joining together, it became a total culture change for this facility. It became a primary initiative for everybody. We developed a lot of different process changes that impact the way we do business, that facilitate our moving people through the system faster.

Kristine Mims, Clinical Director, Emergency Department,
SSM St. Joseph's Health Center

A Good Example of Systems Thinking

Once people realized it would be a primary initiative for everybody in the hospital, people got on board. Excitement began to build. It was the biggest transformation they had ever undertaken.

If we put something in place in any one of our departments without considering the impact that it's going to have on the rest of the hospital, for instance, it's never going to work. It's why, when we started looking at the emergency room thing and how do you reduce waiting time, there wasn't anything that the emergency room could do of themselves. It turned out to be an entire hospital activity. That's the greatest example that I can think of for systems thinking.

Sister Mary Jean Ryan, FSM, RN, President & CEO,
SSM Health Care

We reviewed all of our processes starting from the moment the patient walked in the door to when they were triaged, placed in a room, when the nurse saw them initially, when their labs were drawn, when they were in x-ray. We studied the whole

71

process every step of the way to analyze where our backups were, where we did things well, where we could improve, where we could make the flow better.

Tim Thompson, DO, Emergency Room Director,
SSM St Joseph's Hospital West

The emergency department itself is very dependent upon everybody else in the hospital. We're very dependent on housekeeping and the medical surgical floors and respiratory therapy and radiology and lab. All of our business is dependent upon them being able to be efficient as well.

Kristine Mims, Clinical Director, Emergency Department,
SSM St. Joseph's Health Center

When we started the program, about 30 percent of the patients that would come to us would be seen within 30 seconds or under active care within 30 minutes. We wanted to take that percentage up so that 90 percent or 95 percent of the time we would be successful.

Kevin Kast, President,
SSM St. Joseph's Health Center

GETTING STARTED

The first step in any CQI initiative is to plan. However, to plan reasonably and successfully, one needs data. The emergency room team, made up of members from all departments of the hospital, realized they would have to review all of the emergency room processes starting from the moment the patient walked in the door. They would have to study how patients were triaged, how they were placed in a curtained room in the emergency department, how soon a nurse saw them for the first time, how long it took for labs to be drawn, how long for x-rays to be completed, how long it would take housekeeping to get an upstairs room ready, etc. They had to study the entire process every step of the way to analyze where the back-ups and bottlenecks were and what steps were being done well.

We actually used a time card. The patient clocks in and gets a time stamped right on the card. When they're triaged there's a time stamped for that, when they're placed in a room there's a time for that, when a physician sees them there's a time for that, when they're discharged from the room there's a time for that, or when they are admitted to the room there is time for that. So, we literally analyzed hundreds and hundreds of patients looking for gaps. And we realized initially we have a long time between when the patient signs in and when they are triaged, so we need to streamline in that area. We get that step fine-tuned and we realize we have another gap getting the patient into a room. So, simple things like if we have open rooms and four people walk in at the same time, rather than have all four of those people waiting to be triaged, one would be triaged and the other three would come back to open rooms and they would be triaged in turn in their room.

Tim Thompson, DO, Emergency Room Director,
SSM St Joseph's Hospital West

You really have to look at the turn-around time as the biggest issue for radiology. Before we implemented 30/30, we were looking at a 30- to 45-minute turn-around time for an x-ray—from the time ER physicians ordered the films until the time the films came back and were available to them. After we moved the x-ray room next to the ER, we minimized that to about 15 minutes. The films are shot right here next to the emergency room. They are developed and they are put up for observation by the emergency room physician all in one area. It's close and it's a lot quicker.

Randy Shields, Director Radiology Department,
SSM St. Joseph's Hospital West

DEVELOPING PROTOCOLS

Under the old system, procedures like x-rays and lab work would not be prescribed or started until a physician, face-to-face with the patient, ordered them. What physicians discovered was that almost all patients who come to the ER have a finite range of complaints. In fact, about 30 different situations or treatments cover nearly everyone who enters through the emergency room door. So, treatment protocols—a list of steps to be taken signaled by a certain set of specific symptoms—were developed and approved.

> In order for things to start happening within 30 minutes for patients, we have treatment protocols that have been worked out, established by the nursing staff and physician staff collaboratively. The physicians sign them. For example, if you come into the emergency department with a sprained ankle, the triage nurse assesses you for your complaint and then can order that x-ray of the ankle. She can send you directly to x-ray so that when the physician sees you, you've already been x-rayed. The x-rays are in his hands. He's ready to just look at them and let you go.
>
> *Kristine Mims, Clinical Director, Emergency Department,*
> *SSM St. Joseph's Health Center*

> And say, for instance, you come in and you have chest pains. We all know that a person with chest pains can't sit for a long time. We have a 30-minute window. And what we tell them all the time is: Time is muscle. So, what could I do as a nurse? I could pull that chest pain protocol. I could get an EKG done and get it shown to the physician immediately. I could go ahead and put the patient on some oxygen, put them on a cardiac monitor, and start an IV. I can draw some labs and then start my medicines. I can get nitroglycerin under their tongue to decrease the ischemic injury to the heart. I could give them some morphine for pain. And then some aspirin, and that would just act as a blood thinner. And, hopefully, within a short time, that patient would have decreased anxiety, decreased pain, and less or, hopefully, no damage to the heart. That's the goal that we're looking for.
>
> *Anita Montgomery, RN, ER Team Coordinator,*
> *SSM DePaul Health Center*

THE HOSPITALITY ASSOCIATE

SSM Health Care in their emergency room service also instituted the role of Hospitality Associate. Her job is to see that everyone in the waiting room and throughout the emergency area is doing okay. She is not a nurse, just a friendly person who gives attention and care to everyone in the waiting room. She also frees medical personnel to do medical work.

> We found out that in order to pull 30/30 off, there were certain things that in a very busy clinician's world, the physician or nurse would not have time to do. They would not have time to provide those extra things for body, mind, and spirit, those extra comfort things that people sort of appreciate.
>
> *Brenda Peterson, RN, Patient Access Director,*
> *SSM St. Joseph's Health Center*

> One of the other big things that we initiated was what we call a hospitality person. They're like a hotel concierge. Their whole job is to go around and talk to people and keep people informed on why they are waiting and what's going on. "Are you warm enough? Do you need a blanket?" This is the one thing of all that we did that has been the most valuable.
>
> *Kristine Mims, Clinical Director, Emergency Department,*
> *SSM St. Joseph's Health Center*

> During a very busy period that hospitality associate can help evaluate pain. So, in essence, if a nurse came in and gave somebody something for pain and they are very busy dealing with three or four other patients, the hospitality folks can say things like, "Mrs. Smith, how are you feeling? I know you got something for pain a little while ago. Are you feeling okay now?" If Mrs. Smith is not, the hospitality person is going to find the nurse and to convey what Mrs. Smith is actually feeling right now.
>
> *Brenda Peterson, RN, Patient Access Director,*
> *SSM St. Joseph's Health Center*

> People just love that hospitality person. They're not clinical at all, you know they just fluff and buff everybody.
>
> *Kristine Mims, Clinical Director, Emergency Department,*
> *SSM St. Joseph's Health Center*

On very busy days, the hospitality person helps to clean the beds. If somebody leaves, she goes in and says, "Let me help do this." So, a hospitality associate fills many, many roles, not just that of comforting patients, but also answering questions. Many times in a very busy world, a patient will see the doctor and will forget something. They might say, "Oh, I forgot to tell them that I take this heart medicine." Or "I absolutely forgot to tell him that I've had this pain for longer than just two weeks. I've really had it this length of time." Hospitality goes out and provides that information, so that the nurse or the physician has a complete knowledge of that patient.

Brenda Peterson, RN, Patient Access Director,
SSM St. Joseph's Health Center

HOW IT TURNED OUT

After the first year, the SSM staff were achieving their 30/30 goal about 60 percent of the time, but a year later, when the systems and processes had been smoothed out even more, they had reached 90 percent and have maintained that level for the past two years. They are still working toward 100 percent.

Initially, I must admit, I was one of the biggest naysayers. I said, "They're crazy. I have a problem with this. This is not an urgent care facility. It's not a doc in the box. This is an emergency room. We do important things here, you know. Whoa, we can't do this." But I must admit it's been an excellent, excellent experience.

Kristine Mims, Clinical Director, Emergency Department,
SSM St. Joseph's Health Center

When we started this, we knew we were only achieving the 30-minute time for patients at about the 60 percent mark and now we've been exceeding 90 percent for two years. So, if we take that amount of time-saving for those 65,000 patients that we see on an annual basis, that might be a way to determine how much time we've saved, not only for ourselves but also for the patient.

Maggie Fowler, Vice President of Patient Services,
SSM St. Joseph's Health Center

One of the surprising and delightful benefits of CQI and systems thinking is it does work, as SSM staffers in St. Louis discovered. The whole 30/30 project was an eye-opener, both to systems thinkers and others as it became clear that processes in the entire hospital had to be changed to make the ER improvement successful. PRHI hospitals workers were even more doubtful when they were asked to practice automobile production principles and methods. Their story is in the next chapter.

SOME THINGS TO REMEMBER FROM THIS CHAPTER

✔ An improvement in one department of the hospital, e.g. reducing waiting time in the emergency room, will affect the whole hospital and require every department's support.

✔ The system (or hospital) is made up of subsystems and processes.

✔ A process is a group working together to achieve a single purpose.

✔ When a process—being redesigned and improved—is clearly understood by everyone involved, people can do more than they expected they could.

CHAPTER 8

WHAT WE LEARNED FROM THE TOYOTA PRODUCTION SYSTEM: FOCUS ON THE CUSTOMER/PATIENT

On this unit we had resistance. They said, "What do you mean Toyota production is going to help the Shadyside Hospital?" But when you start tearing apart the principles that they have and how you get to the root of a problem, define it and fix it, you learn how to fix it so that it's never broken again. It's amazing.

Tina Danzuso, RN, Ward Director General Surgery, Shadyside Hospital, PRHI

LEARNING ABOUT QUALITY

Although it may initially seem odd, Pittsburgh hospital staffs learned how to improve their healthcare work from Toyota, the automobile manufacturer. Toyota, noted for its high quality cars, helped develop systems thinking and continual quality improvement as a management system for manufacturing.

In the 1950s American statistician and quality philosopher W. Edwards Deming worked with Toyota and other Japanese companies to help them improve product quality. His ideas, tested and implemented over the next half century, allowed Japan to capture world markets in automobiles and electronic appliances. Dr. Deming said his quality philosophy worked also for delivery of services as well as production of goods.

Dartmouth professor and physician Paul Batalden was the first doctor to recognize the benefits of Dr. Deming's view of systems thinking for hospitals and health care delivery. He attended an early

Deming seminar in the 1980s--the other attendees were ball bearing manufacturers.

As Dr. Batalden began to apply systems thinking to hospitals, he realized that catwalks in auto manufacturing plants over the assembly line made it easy to see the systems and processes as the work moved past. He also realized that Dr. Deming's view of a system which made the customer a part of the system of production was applicable to health care, if hospitals were willing to acknowledge that patients and caregivers were part of the same system.

He began to teach healthcare workers to imagine a catwalk above their hospitals so they could see how their work, frequently in different areas, was connected and how patients and caregivers were part of the same system. The catwalk viewpoint is an excellent approach to seeing systems and processes in hospitals and non-manufacturing plants.

Toyota was among the Japanese companies that first took Deming's ideas to heart.

WHAT DEMING TAUGHT THE JAPANESE

♦ Any organization that provides products and services must view itself as an integrated system, not just a collection of people, machines, and separate departments. All of it must work as one, with a single shared purpose.

♦ Unless all the individuals and departments of an organization share a commitment to a single unifying purpose or aim, there can be no system. Without a single shared purpose, the organization is a collection of individuals each with his or her own agenda and a collection of departments each pursuing its own purpose. A single shared purpose is the only thing that can unite them.

♦ Satisfying and delighting the customer is the only purpose that can unify an organization. In a hospital, that purpose would have to be described as "perfect patient care," or something like that.

♦ Such an organization must include its customers as well as its suppliers as integral parts of the system. In a hospital, this would mean that patients and their families, as well as health insurers, equipment suppliers, food suppliers, pharmacies, and all others who supply things for the hospital, must be treated as integral parts of the hospital's system, not something outside it.

79

◆ Whenever decisions are to be made or changes implemented, they must be based on accurately gathered data. The data must be gathered for that organization. It is useless for one hospital simply to copy what another hospital is doing. For each organization, the facts are almost always different, so the implementation of any improvement will also be different.

◆ Continually improve each product, each service, and each person in the organization. It is the only way to guarantee consistently optimal quality of products and services in health care.

PRHI's CEO, former Treasury Secretary Paul O'Neill, had used the Toyota methods to greatly improve safety and capitalization (800 percent increase) when he was head of Alcoa. So he knew the power of Toyota quality methods.

In the following stories in this chapter, you will see how the people at both PRHI and SSM Health Care grasped and implemented each of these principles that Deming taught the Japanese—how they came to realize that they needed to have a single shared purpose in order to unite their healthcare facilities, how they realized that "perfect patient care" could be their only unifying purpose, how they saw the importance of involving their suppliers and patients in achieving their purpose, how they needed to keep gathering data and make any changes only when enough data has been gathered, and how PRHI trained everyone in the Toyota principles of continual improvement.

The pharmacy story describes how employees, by viewing themselves as customers and suppliers of each other within a process, could help continually improve that process.

The story of the patients sitting uncomfortably half-naked in a hallway waiting for a hospital bed focuses on the need to keep the hospital's shared purpose—perfect patient care—in the forefront of everyone's mind.

In the story of the missing wound dressings and gowns, we see how people trained in the Deming/Toyota principles have developed a new mentality and new tools to initiate in their departments any necessary changes in patient care that help continually improve services.

The Pittsburg medical community was willing to learn these methods because it soon discovered that Toyota's ultimate purpose in making the best automobiles was parallel to their ultimate purpose of delivering optimal healthcare services.

> It's very interesting that the ideal for Toyota and production of cars is our ideal for the delivery of health care, and that ideal is that we deliver (our service or product) one at a time; we meet the patients' (or automobile buyers') needs as uniquely described: on demand, defect-free, waste-free and in an environment that's professionally, emotionally and physically safe for everyone.
>
> *Randall B. Smith, PhD. Associate Dean,*
> *University of Pittsburgh School of Pharmacy*

According to Steven J. Spear, senior fellow at the Institute for Healthcare Improvement, headquartered in Cambridge, Massachusetts, and an expert on applying Toyota's principles to healthcare improvement,

> No organization has fully institutionalized to Toyota's level the ability to [1] design work as experiments, [2] improve work through experiments, [3] share the resulting knowledge through collaborative experimentation, and [4] develop people as experimentalists. But there's reason for optimism... These approaches have been successful when piloted in health care. [1]

A Culture of Continual Improvement and Learning

In the previous chapter SSM leaders described these same methods as building a culture of continual improvement in a hospital system. Students of Dr. Deming guided SSM in their initial efforts.

Dr. Spear also brings an expanded understanding of healthcare problems, the Toyota solution and the efficacy of systems thinking, to hospitals and other organizations.

> The gap...between the U.S. health care system's performance and the skills and intentions of the people who work in it... stem partly from the system's complexity, which creates many opportunities for ambiguity in terms of how an individual's work should be performed and how the work of many individuals should be successfully coordinated into an integrated whole.... Unless everyone is completely clear about the tasks

that must be done, exactly who should be doing them, and just how they should be performed, the potential for error will always be high.

The problem also stems from the way healthcare workers react to ambiguities when they encounter them. Like people in many other industries, they tend to work around problems, meeting patients' immediate needs but not resolving the ambiguities themselves. As a result, people confront "the same problem, every day for years" (as one nurse framed it for me) regularly manifested as inefficiencies and irritations—and occasionally, as catastrophes.

But as industry leaders like Toyota, Alcoa, Southwest Airlines, and Vanguard have demonstrated, it is possible to manage the contributions of dozens, hundreds and even thousands of specialists in such a way that their collective effort not only is capable and reliable in the short term but also improves steadily in the longer term.

In the following pages, PRHI staff and a number of Pittsburgh hospital doctors and nurses testify how they have been learning to apply the four Toyota approaches throughout their hospitals and healthcare facilities. But first they needed to learn Toyota's principles, and become Toyota converts.

REDESIGNING WORK ACCORDING TO PRINCIPLES

A lot of people associate Toyota Production System principles with building cars. In fact, Toyota is really about designing work and doing the work. How do we understand work? How do we improve work? So, it's not just about cars, it's about how we do our work.

Peter Perreiah, Director,
PRHI

Toyota principles are essentially building blocks. They are designed mechanisms about the way work is done. It's not about making fenders, making wheels, and putting seats in cars, or anything like that. It's about work in general. So, the principles apply generically to the way people together working in an organization produce a product, information or service.

David Sharbaugh, Director of Quality Improvement,
Shadyside Hospital, PRHI

A hospital is not a factory, so it is hard to change things overnight. When you are fitting a change process into a very complex environment like a hospital, you have to do this very carefully with people who really know the culture, the workings of the hospital. It's very hard to impose such a framework on a hospital, even though it's worked exquisitely well in other settings.

Karen Wolk Feinstein, Chair & Founder of PRHI,
President Jewish Healthcare Foundation

The first thing we often hear when we talk to people in health care about Toyota is, "Oh, you don't understand. Cars are simple, but health care is very complex." I often chuckle because the average car has about 5,000 parts in it—a little more complex than people realize.

Peter Perreiah, Director,
PRHI

If you look at the products that come from Toyota, they pride themselves on quality and zero errors. Here, it's the same concept. Really, it's taking these tools and techniques and applying them to health care, where the ideal is to have zero errors and the best outcomes. It's not like these ideas are just applicable to a car or to somebody making a car, they are applicable to hospitals. But I really didn't think that to begin with.

I went along with it, went to the program and said, "Okay, I'll just do this because everybody seems to be doing it. I'll try to learn what's going on." And so, I didn't' really go in with an open mind. It was, actually, the application of some of these tools and techniques and some things that occurred here at Allegheny General Hospital in the last 8 to 12 months that made me a believer. I saw outcomes improve and people doing what is right for the patient. So I saw results and that's what proved it.

Connie Cibrone, President & CEO,
Allegheny General Hospital, PRHI

LEARNING TO DO IT BETTER AS YOU DO IT

According to Steven Spear, what sets apart the operations of organizations using Toyota principles "is the way they tightly couple the process of doing work with the process of learning to do it better as its being done."

The Toyota Production System actually gives you a direction about what to change and how to change it. So, it's not a matter of a lot of people sitting in a conference room talking with as much intelligence as they have about a subject and how they can improve it. But it's actually about watching the work and trying to design the process to make it such that you can't fail.

David Sharbaugh, Director of Quality Improvement,
Shadyside Hospital, PRHI

We are proud to derive learning and a systems approach from the principles perfected by Toyota as a place that understands how to constantly improve the ways they meet customer needs across a very complex task and organization. They do it by focusing on core principles and empowering everybody in the organization to act on them through a distinct design.

Kenneth Segel, Former Executive Director,
PRHI

And one of the things about the Toyota production system is that it's really less about projecting from the top the way work is to be done as much as it is on the front line, changing the way work is done by focusing on and observing the hard wiring, and applying these basic design principles to the actual work.

David Sharbaugh, Director of Quality Improvement,
Shadyside Hospital, PRHI

The design principles are what I think is really good about it. They design the waste out of the system instead of trying to squeeze it out. When you are squeezing it you are essentially completely devoid of any sense of understanding what it takes to get the work done. The difference is you can't change the design of work with a real direction in mind by squeezing. When you work with design principles, you spend time seeing and understanding what it takes to do this work successfully.

David Sharbaugh, Director of Quality Improvement,
Shadyside Hospital, PRHI

You fix it so that it's never broken again. It's amazing. And I see a lot of wasted steps that we've done for a lot of years.

Tina Danzuso, RN, Ward Director General Surgery,
Shadyside Hospital, PRHI

A SYSTEM FOR NEVER-ENDING IMPROVEMENT

Once they grasped the principles, they were able to follow in Toyota's footsteps, as it were, in organizing themselves for continual learning, innovation, and improvement.

The main principles of Toyota have to do with how we actually standardize and define the work we do in terms of the content, timing, and sequence. How do we support each member of a system with a supplier and how do we define those relationships? How do we actually define pathways so that the sequence of customer-supplier relationships flows through an organization? Are things defined so that we have a system for improving the actual provision of goods and service?

Peter Perreiah, Director,
PRHI

So, whether you are transporting a patient from a nursing unit to the radiology department or processing trays in the cafeteria, there is application because it's really about the way people

85

are connected to each other along a pathway doing work or providing a service.

David Sharbaugh, Director of Quality Improvement,
Shadyside Hospital, PRHI

Jeffrey K. Liker in his book *The Toyota Way* explains, "Toyota's assumption is that if you make teamwork the foundation of the company, individual performers will give their hearts and souls to make the company successful…. It is about challenging and respecting employees at the same time." [2] There will more about this when we explain O'Neill's philosophy of respecting people in a later chapter. Deming and Toyota principles were also inspiration for the Baldrige National Quality Award. So it is more than building cars.

> When people involved in health care turn their nose up at manufacturing processes, they shouldn't. They are grounded in the scientific principle that we're going to make things perfect. We're going to discover the underlying truth and, at the end of the day, it's much more important that we make defect-free health care to protect human beings than it is that we make defect-free cars. If the door doesn't fit right on a car, that's a customer complaint. If the door doesn't fit right, so to speak, on a health care outcome, then that's a person who may be crippled for the rest of his or her life.
>
> *Cliff Shannon, President, SMC Business Council,*
> *Pittsburgh, PA*

> I compare the challenge of improving the treatment of depression, diabetes and other chronic diseases to the huge leap that manufacturers such as PPG have made in quality. In the 1970s, companies focused on quality control. That meant we checked for defects before the products left the loading dock. Today, good companies focus their quality efforts on their processes to make absolutely sure that the defect never reaches the loading dock. And we're taking that same approach in our plan to address chronic diseases such as diabetes and depression.
>
> *Raymond LeBoeuf, CEO,*
> *PPG Industries*

Refocusing on the patient and what the patient needs is a very powerful tool in our regional initiative to get people back to thinking about where medicine is supposed to start. It's very easy for people to get distracted in the issues of finance or in hospital politics or in competition between each other. When we've been able to refocus people on the goal of the whole endeavor—getting the best possible patient outcomes—people really come together and collaborate to do the best they can to improve patient care. And they share information in the best possible ways.

Geoff Webster, Associate Director,
PRHI

TOYOTA PRINCIPLES IN THE PHARMACY

Serving the patient or customer is the underlying purpose of the Toyota system. Dr. Deming taught that there are many *internal customers* throughout systems, in addition to the ultimate patient or car buyer, called the *external customers*. Whoever provides a product or service to an employee is called an *internal supplier*. As you observe the steps of any process, you can see that every person involved in the process is an internal supplier and has an internal customer. If you are my internal customer, you can tell me how I can best serve you and make your job easier. Dialogue between customer and supplier is one of the best ways to continually improve service. Every process and person has a customer in the supply chain as the pharmacist explains,

> The Toyota Production System principles define a framework in which you can perform your work. It's not like we're making cars in the pharmacy. However, when they talked about supply-chain concepts and customer service, we as a department felt that we were providing exactly the service that nursing needed. "Here, I have sent you the drug, what's the complaint?"

> And we're learning now that service starts with the customer, ultimately the patient. So we now ask, "What does the nurse need to service that customer and what does the pharmacy need to do as a supplier to that customer?"

The Japanese word for signal is *kanban*. Traditionally, a *kanban* is a signal or a card that has information on it that tells you what you need, when you need it, how you need it, where it goes. They have colors, bar codes, and a variety of symbols to give you information about acquiring more of a quantity. It's a single tool we had developed and put all throughout the pharmacy. It took time. The investment up front was significant. However the payoff in the long term was multifactorial. We're reducing the number of times we run out of something. We have more appropriate levels of inventory on the shelf, and anyone that's doing an order or using stock knows when to order and how much to order.

Here is a simple bin available from multiple vendors. On the front is the medication name that is to be stored in here—Lorazapam is an anti-anxiety medication. It tells the brand name and strength and also the order number for when we order from the supplier—the number we use to order that product. And the bin has two sections. The working stock is in the front. When you've used up everything up front and you get to the card, it tells you it's time to order more. So, it doesn't matter who is pulling the medication, whoever uses up the last one— just like at home when you use the last roll of toilet paper—you put another one in there.

Kelley A. Wasicek, R.Ph., Pharmacy Manager,
UPMC Presbyterian Hospital, PRHI

PEOPLE, NOT CARS

In the beginning, I didn't really know what to think about the Toyota Production System and how it was going to be able to make improvements in health care. The most common comment we heard was, "But these are people. They are not cars." Although it's very hard to standardize processes that involve people, after learning what the Toyota Production System was all about, we discovered how it helps you understand your current condition. And there are lots of things that you can improve and can standardize.

Even though we are dealing with patients who are all unique

cases, there are lots of similarities and standard practices. Yet, they have a lot of variation in them; so initially I wasn't sure how it would end up. But I must say, after two years, I am impressed with the job that we have been able to do, and I believe that we can go a lot further in improving the patient care system using these techniques.

Toyota provides a direction. It's not just, "Let's make this better." It's, "Let's try to create continuous flow. Let's try to get work done defect free at a low cost." The Toyota system actually exposes the gap between the current condition and some future improved state. It's that gap that the teacher has to help people see and then understand how they actually create an experiment to close the gap, implement and test it.

Ellesha Miller, RN, Team Leader,
VA Hospital Learning Alliance

HALF NAKED PATIENTS

The following story shows how it takes someone with a fresh perspective and seeing the patient's experience and point of view—to recognize a problem and the need for improvement.

Patients, once they were registered, were sent into a dressing room to change into gowns. Then they were asked to sit in the gowns in a row of chairs in an open hallway until there was a bed available for them. Every day...all the beds were filled up, and so patients would change into gowns and sit in a chair waiting in the hallway. They were sitting in a kind of a flimsy gown, and it wasn't very dignified; it wasn't very nice for them.

Essentially, the patient was being pushed into this hallway where there wasn't a real true connection with another person. So they would pile up in these chairs kind of like inventory items between processes. Only a whole lot worse.

The nurses said that there were times when there were seven people sitting in chairs, and they would get angry and frustrated. They were half naked; it was really a bad scenario.

There happened to be a new physician on the staff up there,

89

and he questioned why patients had to be sitting in these chairs in that condition. We went to the charge nurse and she admitted it was a problem.

She said, "You know, patients complain every day. I always get people yapping about it. But I need them to be ready when I have a bed freed up. I don't know how much work I'm going to have to do in the meantime, so I need them in the chairs ready in their gowns, so that when a bed frees up I can pop them in a bed right away and get the work done."

Part of spending time there and observing the work is that you get to understand what it really takes to get a patient ready—what the nurse is talking about when she says, "I need to get them ready."

Now, the patients, following registration, stay with their family in the waiting room until their bed is available. Only then does the nurse call out, "Please send Mr. Smith back to Bed 8." The secretary escorts the patient, shows them their bed—that was the getting-lost part of the routine for some patients—shows them their bed, saying, "This is where you will go after you change." She takes them to the dressing room to change into a gown. The change in procedure sounds so simple, but for 15 years that that hospital was open, patients sat in chairs half-naked every day. Now they don't.

Will this new practice last? In terms of the sustainability I think the point is that when you actually change the underlying steps of the work system, it's difficult to slip back.

David Sharbaugh, Director of Quality Improvement,
Shadyside Hospital, PRHI

"Slipping back" is always a problem that sabotages improvement efforts. This is an excellent example of how to train the staff to observe a process, discover a problem, and then devise and test a process improvement. Remember, redesigning the work process means that it will be more likely to be standardized until additional opportunities to improve it are seen, studied and tested.

THE MISSING DRESSING AND GOWN

Sometimes it takes a person with a fresh viewpoint to recognize a problem. But Toyota, according to Steven Spear, "teaches people at all levels of an organization to become experimentalists…thereby building exceptionally adaptive and self-renewing organizations."

> We had just taken the dressings off an external incision. Sometimes, when that happens, you pull a little clot or something happens that the incision will drain a little bit. And that's a normal thing, not a big deal. It's just expected that it's going to happen after open-heart surgery. Well, I would come over to the drawer and open it up to get a dressing and to get a clean gown.
>
> Many times, we'll go into the nurse server drawer and we'll find that the needed supplies are not in there. So the nurse will have to go to the supply room, find what is needed, say, two-by-two gauze pads, and then go back and care for the patient.
>
> Well, while I'm in the supply room, somebody calls me and says, "Hey, Pam, could you please help me with this boost?" So I help them to boost this patient.
>
> Well, while I'm boosting, I get a call overhead that says, "Pam, another room needs you stat, right away," so I go running back there and I have a patient who's in excruciating pain, can't wait.
>
> I go get some pain medication and bring it back to him. While I'm doing that I get a call for something else. An hour or so later, I remember, "Oh, I went to get that gown and dressing for the patient down the hall." So I go in there. In the meantime, the gown has a lot more blood and drainage on it so the patient has grabbed napkins, something they've blown their nose on, possibly adding contamination that we can avoid.
>
> *Pam Seigh, RN, Clinical Supervisor,*
> *Allegheny General Hospital, PRHI*

And there's a lot of very simple ways that we can change that kind of situation by looking at how we can design a system so that what the nurse and nursing assistant need is right at the bedside—that they don't have to leave in the middle of a bath.

Deborah Thompson, RN, Quality Trainer,
PRHI

What we're trying to do is make sure that these drawers are re-plenished on a consistent basis, so the nurse never has to leave the room to get what he or she needs.

Deborah Ruckert, Quality Improvement Director,
Allegheny General Hospital, PRHI

I went to the Toyota System Perfecting Patient Care University and we learned a technique to help make care of our patients more efficiently.

Pam Seigh, RN, Clinical Supervisor,
Allegheny General Hospital, PRHI

That means the staff learns to view their work as scientists who collect data, conceive an improvement and test it. That is called the PDSA cycle: Plan, Do, Study, Act.

I learned that we spend a lot of our time walking around doing unnecessary motions and movements and getting unnecessary supplies and looking for things. This takes a lot of our time away from actual care of our patients. One of the things I decid-ed to do to try to help us spend more time in the room with our patients was to develop a system where all of the supplies that the nurse needs, in the amount that she needs, when she needs them and where she needs them, would be available to her.

My system has little organizers and numbers and cards in the drawer that show exactly what should be in the drawer. We also have a specific person who at a specific time replaces the items in the drawer. This gives the nurse and the nurse aide more time with the patient. It also will decrease the amount of stock that we eventually need here on the unit, thereby saving us some money.

Pam Seigh, RN, Clinical Supervisor,
Allegheny General Hospital, PRHI

Spear points out that many of the problems in hospitals—work-arounds, medical mistakes, missed medications, or wrong medications—are shrouded in ambiguity. Someone is *supposed* to be responsible for this procedure, but no one is quite sure who is responsible for each specific aspect of it. Sometimes timing is ambiguous. It is unclear *when* a procedure or action needs to be taken. At other times, the system has not provided specific ways of integrating all the steps of a process. Whenever ambiguity exists over "exactly who is responsible for exactly what, when, and how," Spear says, "eventually a breakdown occurs."

Like many of the improvements made throughout the hospital, Pam Seigh's redesign of the patient's drawers was aimed, as Spear says, "at removing ambiguity and increasing specificity." It included (1) which drawer was to get what put into it, (2) who was responsible for re-supplying the drawers, (3) what signs or signals would be used to initiate the need, and (4) how and when each step would be carried out.

> In my system now, you will be able to open up the drawer and a gown should be there. You open up a drawer and the dressing should be there. I will show you exactly how it works. If I was entering a patient's room and was going to have to change a dressing, I would open up the drawer, I would get the dressing from the drawer, also my little card, called the *kanban* card. It tells us on here the location or the room that it should be in, the drawer that it should be in, where in the drawer it should be, and what it is for. For each four-by-four sponge that is in the drawer there is a card. When I remove the sponge, I put its card in our envelope here, and when the nurse aide is going around replenishing ice and filling up water pitchers at the end of the day, she will see the card and know that she needs to put

a four-by-four into the drawer. And the same thing happens when you remove a gown. Everything is working perfectly. We just needed a little bit of education.

Pam Seigh, RN, Clinical Supervisor,
Allegheny General Hospital, PRHI

Using the Toyota system, I believe, nursing staff has a lot more time with the patients. They are able to spend more quality time with the patients because they are not looking for supplies or waiting for supplies or other things that they may need to do their job.

Ellesha Miller, RN, Team Leader,
VA Hospital Learning Alliance

It is painful–almost unbelievable–to realize that a quality inventory system, absolutely necessary in hospitals to reduce not only waste, but deadly infections, may not already be in place. Missing gowns and dressings or inadequate rubber gloves or inconvenient sterilization stations in a hospital have life-threatening potential. The Toyota inventory system made it possible for hospital staffs to create their own inventory system for these materials and have them always available.

The lesson that these PRHI experimenters took from the Toyota philosophy—focus on the customer/patient—requires the supporting practice of learning everyday on the job how to improve the processes of patient care. That style of learning, seeing waste and mistakes imbedded in traditional, familiar clinical practices, is in turn dependent on the acquired skill of group study and examination of a problem or mistake. Seeing an error or mistake that could endanger a patient, recognizing a step within a process that adds no value for the intended customer, and disclosing the observation without fear of blame, begins the cycle of learning, improvement, and standardization that lifts the hospital's patient care to new levels of quality.

We view errors as opportunities for learning. Rather than blaming individuals, the organization takes corrective actions and distributes knowledge broadly. Learning is a continuous company-wide process as superiors motivate and train subordinates; as predecessors do the same for successors; and as team members at all levels share knowledge with one another.

The Toyota Way, 2001,
Toyota Motor Corporation

Dr. Spear summarizes the potential of the Toyota Production System for improving healthcare institutions:

> The health care system is populated by bright, dedicated, well-intentioned people. They have already demonstrated a capacity to experiment and learn in order to master the knowledge and skills within their disciplines. One can imagine few people better qualified to master the skills and knowledge needed to improve processes that span the boundaries of their disciplines.

Dr. Spear also predicts that if Toyota principles were applied in every American hospital and medical errors were reduced by 90 percent—a reasonable goal we believe—877,000 patients would avoid injury, 39,600 to 88,200 lives would be saved and $15.3 billion to $26.1 billion would be saved annually.

The next chapter tells the story of how these bright and dedicated people developed "new eyes" and learned to use problem-solving processes they learned at Toyota to continually improve familiar hospital routines. Seeing potential problems in old routines is not easy and must be consciously learned.

SOME THINGS TO REMEMBER FROM THIS CHAPTER

✓ An organization that provides goods or services is not a collection of people, machines and separate departments; it is an integrated system and must have an aim.

✓ Everyone in the system must be committed to the aim, which is to serve or supply the needs of a larger system, e.g., customers from society or patients in a hospital.

✓ Focusing on the aim of the system provides unity and purpose, governs decisions and may be used to resolve conflicts.

✓ The people in subsystems and processes of the system are internal customers and suppliers, e.g., the pharmacy supplies medication to nurses for patients.

✓ Satisfying or delighting customers, whether internal or external, is the central focus for the people in the system or organization.

✓ The system includes external customers and suppliers.

✓ All products, services and people must be continually improved.

CHAPTER FOOTNOTES

[1] Steven J. Spear, "Fixing Health Care From the Inside, Today," *Harvard Business Review*, September 2005, p. 91. Spear, has studied PRHI's efforts to transform hospitals. He reports other cases in addition to those we present in this book. He has also written "Decoding the DNA of the Toyota Production System" (*HBR* September 1999) and "Learning to Lead at Toyota" (*HBR* May 2004). We strongly recommend these articles which can be ordered from custserv@hbsp.harvard.edu

[2] Institute of Medicine (2001) *Crossing the Quality Chasm: A New Health System for the 21st Century*. Washington, DC: National Academy of Sciences, p. 1.

CHAPTER 9

WALKING AROUND WITH NEW EYES

It's seeing things differently, seeing through new eyes. I worked here many years, and walking down the hallway I see things today that I didn't see 5, 10, 14 years ago. I think it's because I'm looking at things differently. I'm looking at problems, and when they come up, I have the staff or the nurse find the answer to the problem.... We're now asking the staff to identify the problem and then to come up with the solution.

Tina Danzuso, RN, Ward Director, General Surgery,
Shadyside Hospital, PRHI

Because systems thinking brings about a radical inner transformation, we use metaphors to describe how a person changes as he or she develop these new abilities.

"I (Clare Crawford-Mason) was a nearsighted little girl. I could read words in a book quite easily, but when the teacher wrote words on the chalkboard, they were a blur. I would get the right answers to the problems I copied off the chalkboard, but I had copied the wrong numbers. Finally, at age eleven I got eyeglasses. I felt like I had received new eyes. Everything was cleaner and sharper. I could see leaves on trees and read license numbers on cars! Nothing was blurry or fuzzy anymore!"

Learning systems thinking is like getting a new pair of glasses after having been nearsighted all your life.

We keep saying that systems thinking is a new mindset because you learn to use your mind in a way completely different from the ways you have been using it. And this new mindset also changes your eyes—the very way you see and perceive things. It shifts your vision so that you begin to see clearly things that had always been fuzzy, out of focus or you couldn't see before.

IT TAKES TIME

While Clare's eyeglasses changed her vision instantly, developing systems-thinking eyes takes time and training. It's more like learning to read musical notation or to decipher letters in a language like Greek, Hebrew or Russian that doesn't use our familiar alphabet. After guidance and practice, those little dots and squiggles begin to make sense and reveal their meaning. One day you realize you can read music or a foreign language. What had been impossible before has become easy and natural.

That's what happened to the people at PRHI and SSM Health Care when they say they have "new eyes." After training and practice, they learned to recognize things that had always been there in the hospital unit but that they could never identify clearly before. The essential act here is to see how work gets done and the patient is cared for through a series of processes. These processes can be described and mapped, which makes improvement possible. This chapter is their story about getting new eyes and being able to see "the leaves on trees."

Later in the chapter, in a section called "Learning How to Use New Eyes," hospital staff explain how they learned to ask questions they never asked before and how those questions helped open their new eyes even wider.

In a story about the necessity for hand washing in hospitals, we see how nurses learned to collect data that, when presented clearly, could bring about major changes in behavior.

The chapter ends with a story about a daily search for missing keys that was solved in a few moments when some new eyes looked at the problem. The new answer saved time, money and helped the patients.

TRYING TO EXPLAIN WHAT HAPPENED TO THEM

Of the images the doctors and nurses at SSM and PRHI used to describe the new mindset and inner transformation they developed from studying systems thinking, quality management principles, and the Toyota Production System, the easiest to grasp is getting "new eyes." The new mindset had given them, not simply better eyeglasses to see through old eyes, but truly new eyes. While new eyeglasses may help you to see better what you are used to seeing, new eyes help you to see things you never saw before. So, doctors and nurses and even administrators were walking around the hospital with new eyes. Instead of merely seeing how things are done, they began to see how things could be done differently and better. They even began to predict problems that hadn't occurred because they could see them.

Things like work-arounds and useless steps that used to be carried out automatically as an expected requirement of their jobs were now seen as errors or problems that needed to be eliminated or at least improved.

> Just getting people to think, "Oh, this could be an error," and looking at any situation with open eyes, and not just adapting to it as they had grown accustomed to in the past…. Stopping to think, "You know, this could…cause a problem though it's not now."
>
> *Elaine Hatfield, MPM, Clinical Operations Officer,*
> *LifeCare Hospitals of Pittsburgh, PRHI*

> To have eyes that see differently and eyes that see each problem as an opportunity to be solved, and to understand how we can literally solve specific problems and make specific improvements quickly.
>
> *Kenneth Segel, Former Executive Director,*
> *PRHI*

> That one skill, all in itself, will change the way you think about your work.
>
> *Tami Merryman, RN, Vice President, Patient Care Services,*
> *Shadyside Hospital, PRHI*

> I see my work environment differently now than I saw it several years ago. And I think it is important for us to understand how our work is being done. It's really the prime consideration, because once we understand that—that the way we do our work affects the outcomes that we have, affects our patients—then we understand that we can measure how well we do our work

99

so that we can make a change in it, then see whether it's better or worse. This is a very powerful concept.

Michael H. Culig, MD, Cardiothoracic Surgeon,
West Penn Hospital, PRHI

LEARNING HOW TO RECOGNIZE PROBLEMS

Over the past twenty years here, I have been a direct front-line traditional head nurse, supervisor, and clinical director. I've had hundreds of nurses who have worked for me, and I always thought I did a really good job. I cared about the work environment in which they worked, I understood their problems, and I cared about my patients.

But, you know what? During the past five years, you learn a lot actually working in the shoes of your employee—working beside the person who passes out the linens in the morning, seeing how difficult it is for a nurse when they need to go and get a syringe for a patient out of the medication drawer and it's not there, or how difficult it may be for the fellow who brings up the supplies who has to get five separate keys to put away dressings. That stuff doesn't make any sense.

But I just assumed that was very normal. I think you kind of get used to it. Until I went and observed minute by minute and followed those different disciplines—who all provide care to the patient, maybe not directly but indirectly—I became more learned, I would say, in understanding. Sometimes we have difficult processes to work in.

Susan Christie Martin, RN, Director, Nursing Support Services,
Shadyside Hospital, PRHI

There is a sense that part of our work is to work around problems, so one of the very early difficulties we had on the learning line was that nurses didn't recognize their problems—that they're the ones who are supposed to say, "This isn't working" or "I'm having a problem with that." They had a hard time recognizing a problem because they dealt with it every day by working around it. It turned out that what they had to do—the heroic effort to actually get through their day with many work-arounds—they considered that the work of health care.

> *David Sharbaugh, Director of Quality Improvement,*
> *Shadyside Hospital, PRHI*

LEARNING HOW TO USE "NEW EYES"

Doing observations, measuring and collecting data are all important new eyes skills. And they must be learned and practiced. So, developing new eyes requires training.

> I think that the most important aspect of this way of thinking is to be able to sit back and watch analytically—to *learn* how to watch analytically and to spend the time doing it. That is a skill that, certainly, every physician can develop.
>
> *Michael H. Culig, MD, Cardiothoracic Surgeon,*
> *West Penn Hospital, PRHI*

> It's all about looking. Does the patient get the medicine when they need it? Do they have the right medicine at the closest time? I've been involved in looking at: How do we insure supplies are there? How do we insure that we have time to do the right things for patients?
>
> *Deborah Thompson, RN, Quality Trainer,*
> *PRHI*

> Waste is everywhere. To see it requires a trained eye that is developed over time. But I firmly believe, if there's no other message that gets out to healthcare leadership than this, "Get out of your chair. Get out to your departments and watch what's happening. Because you will be amazed at what you think is happening versus what's really happening." And so, it's the trained eye. Waste is everywhere but you have to know how to look for it.
>
> *Tami Merryman, RN, Vice President, Patient Care Services,*
> *Shadyside Hospital, PRHI*

How New Eyes Help Effect Change

First, with any of these initiatives, you have to go in and understand a current condition—what is actually occurring today. So, we spend a lot of time doing what we call observations—going around, observing nurses, nurse aides, and others—to really understand the work that's being performed on this unit.

Deborah Ruckert, Quality Improvement Director,
Allegheny General Hospital, PRHI

One of the things that were talked about was improving our hand washing compliance. It's sad to say but in health care today people don't wash their hands like they should. I can remember sitting in this room and having several of my esteemed physician colleagues swear up and down, "We all wash our hands. We never not do that. I can't believe anyone would accuse us of such inappropriate behavior."

I just sat there and I listened and I said to myself, "Okay. Yeah. Sure. All right."

Then we went out and trained the infection-control nurses to do observations on hand washing. And our first report was that 32 percent of the physicians wash their hands.

It's a different tone in a meeting when you have your esteemed leader saying, "You're all crazy," and when you go back and you say, "Well, you know, we just happened to go out and look. We observed 18 physicians and six of them wash their hands." And they can't refute it. They can't say, "Well you know..." Then they get all stammering and stuttering about the real facts as if to say, "Just don't confuse my perceptions with facts, you're screwing me up here."

So, did I ever know the magnitude of those issues without looking? If someone were to say to me, "Do you think everybody in your hospital washes your hands?" I'd say, "No, I don't. I'm not stupid. I wasn't born yesterday." But if they asked me, "How many did wash their hands?" Oh, I'd be guessing.

Now, I don't guess. It's the difference between thinking you know what goes on and really knowing, and knowing where to go to address it.

> *Tami Merryman, RN, Vice President, Patient Care Services,*
> *Shadyside Hospital, PRHI*

IDENTIFYING ERRORS

You have to see the errors before you can eliminate them. You have to accept that they are, in fact, errors. Business as usual has no place in systems thinking.

> Just two weeks ago, we all ended up swarming the lab and swarming the emergency department to say, "What can we do in these areas to make things better? And help them learn the eye." So, it's reinforcement. It's a process of working with them side by side.
>
> *Tami Merryman, RN, Vice President, Patient Care Services,*
> *Shadyside Hospital, PRHI*

> The pharmacist had about 150 prescriptions that he received during the day, and all but two of them needed follow-up before he could fill them.
>
> In common practice the pharmacist doesn't see that as an error. He sees it as work.
>
> Most people would say the error occurs when the patient gets the wrong medication.
>
> In systems thinking, when a pharmacist has to go back to find out what the intended communication was, that's an error.
>
> *Paul O'Neill, former U.S. Treasury Secretary,*
> *Former CEO, PRHI*

> Ph.D. pharmacists who man phone lines to intervene with the physicians. This is a significant waste of time.

Those pharmacists could be interacting with patients, doing evaluations and histories, doing education, doing those kinds things that enhance patient safety.

JoAnn V. Narduzzi, MD, Ph.D., VP of Academic Affairs,
Pittsburgh Mercy Health System, PRHI

UNNOTICED ERRORS

Error occurs everywhere, unnoticed, until someone using new eyes notices it. The error could be as simple as a lock and key. We followed nurses minute by minute, shift by shift, for several days and we found a nurse was wasting time looking for a key. And so today each nurse, when he or she comes on the shift, gets her own set of keys. So there's no waste, there's no one running around looking for a key. But most important, the patient is getting what he or she needs right away.

Tina Danzuso, RN, Ward Director, General Surgery,
Shadyside Hospital, PRHI

UNEXPECTED SAVINGS

The keys save 15 minutes each shift, three shifts a day. Over a year, the hospital saves more than 11 days of nurse time on one ward because of one observation.

How you learn is simply going, looking and seeing, solving the problem, trying a solution, changing that solution. And if it doesn't work, trying another solution.

Deborah Thompson, RN, Quality Trainer,
PRHI

It is important to remember that people do not acquire new eyes by willing it or wishing it or by reading about it. New vision requires training and reinforcement. You can't simply invite a group of people into a room and ask them to redesign a certain process. Such a group, if they are to succeed in truly improving a process, must have proficiency in several systems-thinking skills, such as how to do observations, how to collect data, how to measure and record results, how to make flowcharts, and how to carry out the Plan-Do-Check-Act (PDCA) cycle.

Also, the people at PRHI and SSM Health Care discovered that new eyes were best used in teams and that teams were most successful when they shared data and discoveries, which is the theme of the next chapter.

Some Things to Remember From This Chapter

✓ New eyes emerge from seeing the hospital as a system and a new belief that improvements can be made by redesigning how work is done.

✓ New eyes see the workplace from a different perspective, e.g., does this help the patient? Could it be simpler?

✓ New eyes continually see new problems and possibilities for improvement.

✓ New eyes see formerly unnoticed interactions among people and formerly ignored connections between events.

✓ When new eyes look at the workplace culture and processes, they provoke questions about tradition and habits.

✓ New eyes see latent errors.

CHAPTER 10

HOW WE LEARNED TO COOPERATE AND SHARE DATA

I think physicians are surprised sometimes. They think that their practice is relatively the same as other peers. When they find out by sharing that there's differences in length of stay, or there's differences in a procedural pack that they use, or something else, it's eye opening. And it causes them to think in terms of "Well, maybe there is a better way." But the sharing is not done in a punitive or a negative fashion.

Paula Friedman, Vice President, Systems Improvement
SSM Health Care

A NEW REALIZATION

A number of new realizations occur when people across an organization begin to practice systems thinking. Among the most pleasant of these awarenesses is that *cooperation begins to replace competition* and *mutual trust replaces fear*. It is nothing less than an astonishing shift from a win/lose mentality to a win/win mentality.

Americans rarely think about the drawbacks of competition and competitiveness. Most of us have been taught in school, in sports, in families, and especially at work that competitiveness is the winning stance. However, what we are slow to acknowledge about a competitive spirit is that it can produce destructive effects as well, especially within an organization. For example, it can generate rivalry, secrecy, deception, resentment, mistrust, criticism, conflicting goals, unintended outcomes and financial loss, as well as diminished self-esteem in the losers. In a competitive framework, there are always losers.

The cooperative framework of systems thinking ushers in a spread of contrasting benefits. Instead of rivalry, cooperation generates teamwork.

Instead of secrecy, people freely share data and information. Instead of deception, there is honesty and truth, instead of resentment, mutual support and instead of mistrust, openness. Instead of blaming someone, we design improvements so no one can make mistakes. Instead of conflicting goals, there is commitment to a single, shared purpose, instead of losers, all share the victory, and instead of financial loss, the pie grows bigger.

Dr. W. Edwards Deming said without cooperation there can be no true system, only competing individuals and departments and labor and management on opposite teams.

In systems thinking, any change that truly improves the system must be based on accurately gathered data. In a competitive organization, important or damaging data is often hidden, disguised, shared piecemeal, and often in a distorted form, all designed to make the holder of the data look "good."

In contrast, in a cooperative organization, data is openly and honestly shared as an essential foundation of genuine transformation.

Both healthcare systems we studied quickly recognized the power of shared data and created systems among their facilities for gathering, collating, and disseminating research data, so that all facilities could use this data to help design improvements in their procedures and processes.

In this chapter, you will read how the sharing of data among PRHI institutions helped to significantly lower cardiac by-pass operation mortality, and taught cardiac surgeons and nurses how to design a perfect patient discharge.

COOPERATIVE-COMPETING HOSPITALS

The Pittsburgh Regional Healthcare Initiative is a system of more than 41 hospitals, while SSM Health Care is made up of 20 hospitals and two long-term care facilities. Within each system, the hospitals cooperate with one another and frequently gather together to share data and knowledge. However, the PRHI hospitals also compete with each other for patients.

In Pittsburgh, an individual cardiac surgeon may see 200 patients a year. The hospitals together will see 6,000. By sharing, everyone gets much more information in the same amount of time, so improvements can be made faster.

Hospitals need long-term research to pinpoint long-term problems. They need real-time data to solve immediate problems. The cooperative system replaces each doctor's experience with every doctor's experience. So, people coming to team meetings on, say, cardiac surgery can learn from data gathered from thousands of operations.

Sharing Data

> All the hospitals in the area now have an opportunity to share. When we had our own quality and risk management program, we were doing things our way. We really didn't have an opportunity to share our experiences with other hospitals, to ask "How do you manage this issue? What do your doctors do? How do you respond to this problem?" So, we were actually in our own little silo. Now that we have 40-some hospitals in PRHI, we are doing the same kinds of things together. We have regional meetings, we share our experiences, we learn from one another, so that we don't have to go through the same kind of lessons as if we were doing this just by ourselves. The information sharing part of the PRHI, to me, is the most exciting part.
>
> *JoAnn V. Narduzzi, MD, Ph.D., VP of Academic Affairs,*
> *Pittsburgh Mercy Health System, PRHI*

When we began there were many naysayers. Some said it was not possible. With government regulations about information control, we simply can't do this job because we are under the privacy considerations. Other people said you couldn't do this because the medical community sees information as a competitive weapon. They won't agree to come together to create this information for human value, for individual human beings.

The Pittsburgh Health Information Network put the lie to all of that. With the help and assistance and initiative of companies like PPG, the employer, the insurance companies, the health care systems and the individual doctors, we mowed down all of those excuses as to why we can't do it. In a few weeks, this new initiative would begin providing information directly to individual doctors that makes it possible for them to know what needs to be done and to have the information in a timely way.

Paul O'Neill, former U.S. Treasury Secretary,
Former CEO of PRHI

CREATING THE STRUCTURE FOR SHARING

What we've done is create an infrastructure for people to share data and share learning. We've created the capacity to do some analysis on information that people never had before. But, more importantly, what that does is focus them back on each patient, one at a time.

Geoff Webster, Associate Director,
PRHI

We formed task forces. We said, "All right, let's get a member from all these different organizations to sit in a room together and figure out whether this is really a barrier. Let's get the facts straight." And this has been a very exciting process, in trying to put together this information network, in watching how quickly those barriers have collapsed when we have a goal that we know is worth working for, and when everybody who has something to gain from it is involved in figuring out exactly what the problem is. We found solutions left and right.

Deborah Thompson, RN, Quality Trainer,
PRHI

PRHI brings us together as a region, has us share in understanding the data, then sends us back to our institutions, and empowers us to go to work to solve the problems. And they provide the tools. So this is not PRHI coming into our hospital and fixing it. This is PRHI empowering us, based upon regional information, to go back and fix it ourselves.

Richard Shannon, MD, Chairman, Department of Medicine,
Allegheny General Hospital, PRHI

WHAT PHYSICIANS DISCOVERED THROUGH SHARING

Surprisingly, we found that physicians do come to our meetings. They participate in the collaborative because of the information that we provide. We provide data cleanly and succinctly. We provide the sources of the information and we report performance on a relative scale without embarrassing individual physicians, or pointing out how Physician A is better than Physician B. Rather, we point out what Physician A is doing well and how we all can learn from it. And that has been motivating for the physicians.

Paula Friedman, Vice President, Systems Improvement,
SSM Health Care

When we can show them that using an insulin protocol or using a Heparin protocol or using an order set for post-op care or admission diagnosis actually makes it easier to take care of the patients and shows benefits to the patients. When we can show them the data, that these patients have better outcome, they buy into it. Because physicians basically want to do what's right for the patient.

Paul Convery, MD, Chief Medical Officer
SSM Health Care/St. Louis

Data is very important in convincing people that these different procedures and approaches are worthwhile. And making early successes is incredibly important to convince physicians. Maybe in picking a topic where it's almost certain that you will make successes, so that people can believe it, the philosophy and the action that you take actually will have a positive effect on patient care.

Andrew Kosseff, MD, Director, Clinical Systems Improvement
SSM Health Care

If we find out another hospital is performing better in how they manage heart attacks or myocardial infarction, we can go to that hospital and ask, "What are you doing differently?" Then we can reanalyze what we're doing ourselves and we can use some of the information and some of the best practices that they use there, adopting them in our own hospital to do a better job ourselves.

Kevin Johnson, MD, VP for Medical Affairs,
SSM DePaul Health Center

CARDIAC CARE EXAMPLE

In southwestern Pennsylvania there are 13 open-heart programs. Now, some people say there are more open-heart programs than there are Jiffy Lubes. The Pittsburgh Regional Health Initiative brought all the 13 programs together about three years ago. Participants gathered the data from all the programs and shared it in a very open and safe environment, so that an institution such as ours could learn from other institutions what the best practices were.

Richard Shannon, MD, Chairman, Department of Medicine,
Allegheny General Hospital, PRHI

The busiest cardio-thoracic surgeon in the region may do 200 cases in a year. Of those 200 cases, four people will die. Compared to the region where there are 6,000 cases and 120 of them die, there is a lot better opportunity to leverage this sharing of knowledge in order to understand what is happening to their patients.

Dennis Schilling, Clinical Coordinator,
PRHI

The average mortality in southwestern Pennsylvania from a cardiac surgical bypass procedure is about 2.3 percent. We can reduce that another 25 percent by doing four things. First, the uniform use of an aspirin prior to surgery, that costs about 3 cents. Second, the uniform use of beta-adrenergic blocking agents during the induction of anesthesia, which costs about 50 cents. Third, the uniform use of the internal mammary artery as a bypass graft, which costs nothing. And, fourth, the uniform measurements of the blood hematocrit during the bypass operation. In our regional cardiac working group meeting, we recently discovered that, in fact, our mortality is declining, that our use of these four interventions is increasing, and that if we continue along that track further improvements in the outcomes can occur.

Richard Shannon, MD, Chairman, Department of Medicine,
Allegheny General Hospital, PRHI

These are four things that aren't particularly expensive and are very doable. But we need to lay them out there as clearly defined decisions that have to be made over the course of care, whenever a patient comes in for coronary artery bypass surgery. Clinicians make hundreds of decisions on every case going to surgery, in surgery, and immediately following surgery. These are just four things that we're highlighting as clear decisions that have to be made or not made. There is no way that anyone can say if someone made an active decision to use or not to use aspirin before surgery. All we know is that a patient received it or did not receive it. This is the same kind of blame-free assessment that a surgeon could make too: I understand that my patients that received aspirin appear to be doing better.

Dennis Schilling, Clinical Coordinator,
PRHI

We wouldn't be doing this sharing and attempting to change our behavior and the behavior of other surgeons in our institutions if we didn't have the data that support it. Whereas, before, I was not as conscious of the fact that it was necessary for a patient to be on aspirin to within several days of coronary bypass surgery. Now I am convinced that that is the case. The data is there.

Michael H. Culig, MD, Cardiothoracic Surgeon,
West Penn Hospital, PRHI

Individually, we would have never come across that data ourselves. Collectively, by sharing the information, we now have the opportunity to embark upon those kinds of collective and collaborative efforts.

Richard Shannon, MD, Chairman, Department of Medicine,
Allegheny General Hospital, PRHI

I think that there's a sea change going on in the way that we practice medicine. And again, because the consequences of our personal actions can be so devastating to the patient, we tend to practice the way that we were taught and the way that we're comfortable with.

Michael H. Culig, MD, Cardiothoracic Surgeon,
West Penn Hospital, PRHI

THE READMISSION RATE

The next challenge came in questioning the readmission rate following cardiac surgery. The answer was disturbing and offered an opportunity to practice continual improvement.

To have survived a major operation, not only survived it, but survived it to be able to be discharged from a hospital, with a 20 percent chance of having to return in the next 30 days, is astonishing. Worse yet was the observation that half of those readmissions occurred within the first 96 hours. "So I'm (as a patient) going to leave today and there is a 10 percent chance I'll be back within the next four days?" That really suggested to us that there's something in the process of care during the last days prior to discharge that must be fixed.

Richard Shannon, MD, Chairman, Department of Medicine,
Allegheny General Hospital, PRHI

Unfortunately, what we found was that a lot of the time a cardiac surgeon, for instance, will do a procedure and he will never know whether or not that person got readmitted to the hospital. There were many cardiac surgeons in the region that thought that the readmission rate was 5 percent or 6 percent. Turned out to be 17 percent for the region on average. And that's because a lot of people were going back to a different institution or a different doctor when they got sick again.

Geoff Webster, Associate Director,
PRHI

So, the first thing we asked was, "What are the factors that cause people to be readmitted?" They turn out to be infections.

They turn out to be atrial fibrillation, an irregular heart rate. And they turn out to be the development of heart failure due to the fluid overload.

Many patients don't know how to clean their wound because the wound is cleaned for them in the hospital. Unless we educate the patient and their families and provide them with the materials to clean the wound, it would be highly unlikely we would be able to eradicate these infections.

Teaching them these very simple measures, creating a standard discharge format, which makes sure that there's a checklist that we go through that every patient has the proper information, affords us the opportunity to create what we call the perfect discharge. And the perfect discharge we believe will lead to the elimination of readmissions.

Richard Shannon, MD, Chairman, Department of Medicine,
Allegheny General Hospital, PRHI

Now, when the patient comes on the unit, we begin to educate them about the care process—from the time they hit our unit through discharge—rather than waiting until discharge, and then giving them a barrage of information.

Deborah Ruckert, Quality Improvement Director,
Allegheny General Hospital, PRHI

Collecting and sharing data is the first step in predicting what a system will do, whether a single hospital or groups of hospitals such as PRHI and SSM Health Care. As staff in these hospitals used their new eyes and practiced applying the methods of Toyota and CQI, they began to become systems thinkers. They learned to make observations and gather data (facts, statistics, or descriptive information) about slow, troubled or ineffectual processes.

The aim of data gathering is to characterize or measure the performance of processes used in delivery of clinical care. With the information derived from an analysis of data, a team of workers should then be able to answer "who," "what," "when," "where" and "how-many" questions about the process. Such information makes possible an accurate description of the process and its drawbacks, which, in turn, offers possible approaches to improvement, e.g., measuring to be sure improvements actually are improvements.

Decisions about organizing work or processes in hospitals have traditionally been based on habit, conventional wisdom, or intuition. That is no longer effective in a modern hospital. Such decisions require systems thinking.

> So many things are measured. There are so many piles of information. Our managers and department leaders need to figure out how we can synthesize [data] down to the vital [information]. To prioritize information, not just loads and loads of data. How can you turn [data] into useable information that makes a difference in how you are delivering care and providing services day in and day out.
>
> *Paula Friedman, Vice President, Systems Improvement,*
> *SSM Health Care*

FIVE LEVELS OF LEARNING

Systems educator Russell Ackoff and W. Edwards Deming agree that there are five levels of learning—data, information, knowledge, understanding, and wisdom.

Data are collections of symbols—numbers or letters that, by themselves, don't mean all that much. *Information* is data that has been ordered and processed into something that can be understood or grasped. *Knowledge* is information that can be used to do or create or modify something. Knowledge tells us *how* to do something. *Understanding* explains *why* we do something. *Wisdom* tells us *when* and *where* to use or apply our knowledge and understanding. Ideally, a systems thinker should be able to use all these levels of learning.

Most formal education is about data and information. Relatively few people ever go beyond information to acquire knowledge; only some of those few get understanding; and maybe a handful attain wisdom.

Dr. Ackoff warns, "Until managers take into account the systemic nature of their organizations, most of their efforts to improve their performance are doomed to failure."

In the past, companies viewed as machines or as organisms could be run with knowledge. We only had to know *how*. Today, to run a company as a social system, we have to know *why*. We need understanding and wisdom.

Some Things to Remember From This Chapter

✓ Cooperation and data are two essential aspects of systems thinking.

✓ Working at cross-purposes or promoting a win/lose mentality between people or departments will sabotage improvement and interferes with collection of good data.

✓ A cooperative culture is the basic environment for producing improving goods, services and joy in work.

✓ Data allow decisions to be made on facts.

✓ Data include facts, statistics or descriptive information about work and processes.

✓ Decisions about organizing work or processes in hospitals can no longer be based on habit, conventional wisdom or intuition.

✓ Analyzing data answers questions about work and processes and can identify which changes are actually improvements.

CHAPTER 11

HOW WE BECAME SYSTEMS THINKERS

The health system in this country and around the world has been based on individual excellence. And we have, arguably, the best trained physicians and nurses in the world—all giving their individual very best to do the best job. In a complex environment like health care, everybody doing his or her very best obviously is not good enough. We have to have a systems approach to be able to tie all of this together.

Paul Convery, MD, Chief Medical Officer
SSM Health Care/St. Louis

The heart of what staffs at PRHI and SSM Health Care learned in their training from Toyota or with CQI (Continuous Quality Improvement) training, is a new mindset called *systems thinking*. It is this revolutionary mindset that allowed and enabled these healthcare professionals to improve their facilities.

Essentially, systems thinking allows people to see a bigger picture—to see the whole rather than just pieces or parts of it. Systems thinking treats the "whole" as more than the sum of its parts. The parts of the system are the people and the machines in it. Paradoxically, the "whole" they learn to see is the product of the interaction of the parts—including all those intangible and invisible exchanges and interactions of the people in the system. They learn to see many things they never saw before.

They learn that the quality of the whole system is created by how well all the parts work together. If all the parts are to work together effectively and efficiently, they must agree on a shared aim or purpose for the system. In the case of a hospital, the only aim large enough that can unify all the disparate parts of a healthcare system is perfect or *continually improving patient care.*

117

Making this transition to big-picture thinking is very difficult in most American organizations, because our culture has taught us to emphasize individual initiative rather than team effort, short-term outlook rather than long-range aims and continual improvement, and to rely on single-event thinking rather than systems thinking.

It is important to realize, that systems thinking is not quite American or Western.

Americans like to say, "If it ain't broke, don't fix it." They like to avoid problems. In direct contrast, systems thinking tells you to continually ferret out problems to solve, discover ways to fix them, and experiment with better ways to do things. The systems thinker understands that striving for continual improvement means the job is never done.

Americans like to find someone to blame whenever something goes wrong. In contrast, studies have found that more than 90 percent of all problems have their source in faulty procedures and can't be traced to a single individual. So, systems thinking says, "Rather than look for someone to blame, let's fix the process so that what went wrong can't ever go wrong again."

Americans are task-oriented. They like to say, "Tell me what I'm supposed to do and I'll get it done. Don't bother me with what others have to do." A systems thinker says, "I can't really do a good job unless I know how what I do fits with what everyone else is doing."

Americans and we authors are Americans still learning to recognize and temper these limiting beliefs like to think they are individually self-sufficient. We say we know how to do our job and don't need or have time to learn anything more. System thinkers say that learning how to redesign processes to make them ever more efficient and effective requires that everyone keep learning continually.

Finally, Americans seem to love the solitary brave hero, the one valiant man or woman who steps into a chaotic problem and saves the day. We were all brought up on superhuman comic book heroes like Superman, Spiderman, and the Lone Ranger. Even in our national mythology, it is always the solitary man--Paul Bunyan, Johnny Appleseed, or Daniel Boone--who is our gallant hero. We tend to forget that our American villages and towns were built by the dedicated teamwork and devoted cooperation of thousands of unsung pioneer men and women. Instead, we focus on the outstanding individual genius of a certain few—like George Washington, Thomas Jefferson, or Benjamin Franklin. It may be the flip side of finding someone to blame—the lone person who saved the day.

In hospitals and health care, we also like to focus on the individual surgeon or physician who seems to perform miracles. However, improvement of a hospital system doesn't work that way. It requires giving up the idea that one amazing individual is going to come in and save the day using "command and control" management. True healing requires the enlightened cooperation of everyone. And that calls for more than coming to work and doing your best. Independent individuals doing their personal best without systems knowledge have actually helped make hospitals malfunction as badly as they do.

In the two hospital systems we studied, the healing process required giving up both "command and control" management and the "individual excellence" approach. Instead, people adapted to the systems mindset, which focuses on cooperation and teamwork to achieve a shared purpose. The systems-thinking mindset led them to making healthcare procedures better and better in a never-ending cycle of improvements.

> Most of us of my age and even…younger grew up or were trained in a method called command and control. I would command you to do something, you would do it, and therefore I would have control. What we are now trying to say is no one individual has the ability to direct people in a way that's meaningful around everything that has to do with health care. It's just absolutely impossible. What would it be like if we said instead, "I'm not going to command you to do this. What I am going to do is give you the educational things that you need to be able to identify some things that we can work on and some ways that we can work together. Then, what I will also do is give you the freedom to make the changes you need to make. And if you make a mistake while we're doing this, it's not going to be your fault. It's the fault of the process. And what we

will learn from your failure is greater than any of the successes that we might have."

Sister Mary Jean Ryan, FSM, RN, President & CEO,
SSM Health Care

We're constantly testing the limits and the balance between what we're doing as a system and what individual facilities are doing. For the most part, I think we've reached a very comfortable balance, recognizing we're a large system. As administrators of the larger system, we have to set the direction and the parameters, but health care is truly delivered on a local basis. So, we allow the system to become self-organizing to meet the needs of the local community.

William P. Thompson, Senior Vice President,
Strategic Development, SSM Health Care

I think what systems thinking says is that you can't do one thing in isolation without knowing that it's going to impact all other things. So, if we set out a policy, thinking that it's the right thing to do without checking out the implications of it or knowing the things that could go wrong, it's really the way that health care has gotten to be in the mess that it's in. It's because we have never looked at what are all the things that could go wrong if we do this.

Sister Mary Jean Ryan, FSM, RN, President & CEO,
SSM Health Care

The crisis in American health care is the failure to see how the parts connect to the final solution. Seeing those connections will improve the outcomes for patients dramatically, as well as reduce the cost.

Peter Perreiah, Director,
PRHI

EVERY SYSTEM MUST HAVE A SHARED FOCUS

A system first comes into existence when all of the parts of that system share a single purpose or aim. Until then, it is not a true system, but merely a collection of parts. In a mechanical system, like an automobile, the parts are assembled for a single purpose, to provide transportation. In a complex social organization like a hospital, the system is made up of people as well as machines. So, all of the people involved must agree on a universally shared purpose, otherwise the employees, departments, equipment, and materials that make up that organization form no true system, only a collection of different parts each with its own agenda. PRHI and SSM Health Care became true systems when each agreed to have everyone pursuing the same, shared purpose, namely *improving patient care*. After all, only when an organization has a clear purpose can anyone tell whether or not a change in policy, procedure, process, or practice is an improvement. And only a clear purpose can allow the people to identify faulty processes.

> The system should be centered on patient needs and have all the different players do their best to resolve those needs. Our healthcare system in the United States now is not working that way. Each segment, each player is seeing only their own angle and not the entire process. And if there are no common rules and if there is no common purpose and there is no commonly agreed upon requirement, it's impossible to make this process efficient.
>
> *Alberto Colombi, MD, Chief Medical Officer,*
> *PPG Industries*

> What a systems approach has allowed us to do is articulate some very explicit goals and expectations, starting with our mission statement: "Through our exceptional health care services we reveal the healing presence of God."
>
> We have created a series of values around stewardship and justice and respect and quality. That has been clearly articulated and communicated.
>
> *William P. Thompson, Senior Vice President,*
> *Strategic Development, SSM Health Care*

> So much of health care has been task-oriented. It's fixing this issue, it's addressing this particular problem without under-

standing the context of the whole patient view—the patient's perspective.

Paula Friedman, Vice President, Systems Improvement,
SSM Health Care

PROCESSES AND SUBSYSTEMS: THE BUILDING BLOCKS

A complex system such as a hospital is made up of many subsystems, such as the emergency department, intensive care units, surgery, x-ray, pharmacy, admissions, purchasing, billing, housekeeping, etc. Each subsystem is made up of many different processes, that is, common procedures that require the interaction of people and machines in a sequence of steps.

For example, the delivery of medication to a patient is a process that involves a number of departments and people, the doctor who writes the prescription, the pharmacist who fills it, the person who fills the medication carts with prescriptions for every patient on a certain unit, the person who checks to see that each medication is correct, and the person who delivers the medication to the patient's room and administers it. The secret of continual quality improvement in a system is the continual improvement of each process in the system.

> There was never this goal of saying we have this thing called a process and we want to improve it. Instead everybody had a step in the process and that was his or her little piece. A process is basically a system, but if you only know one piece of it, you're never going to be able to fix the process.
>
> *Sister Mary Jean Ryan, FSM, RN, President & CEO,*
> *SSM Health Care*

> One of the first things we taught folks is that process has often cut across individual departments. And in fact most of the problems in delivery of care are not necessarily within the department but in the hand-offs between departments. So we started cross-functional groups. And we have discovered a lot of people with great creativity and imagination and ability to help us improve our macro systems, our macro processes.
>
> *William P. Thompson, Senior Vice President,*
> *Strategic Development, SSM Health Care*

MEETING RESISTANCE TO SYSTEMS THINKING

The difficulty in bringing systems thinking into a hospital is that it requires that you begin to look at everything you do—and everything others do—in a new way. And most people don't like that. It is difficult to get off automatic pilot and develop awareness. People resist.

> Typically, doctors are very supportive once they find out what we are doing. We didn't go as far as fast with the doctors as we would have liked. It's very important, for example, to modify doctor behavior regarding precaution compliance (washing hands and sterile clothes) to reduce the risk of transmission of pathogens. Some of our doctors, but not all, got excellent systems thinking training and attended orientation sessions. After two years, we've built the relationships throughout the services, so that we now have doctors training other doctors. These doctors are now engaged in thinking about potential problems with their patients, looking at different aspects of prevention, and reducing patient risk. For example, surgeons are thinking about their high-risk patients, asking if there are any additional precautions they can take, say, before surgery, to lower the risk of patients contracting an infection.
>
> We wish we knew how to systematically get to the doctors and motivate them to devote their time, their energy, and their leadership skills to persuade their peers to focus on these problems. We are gaining traction now. I think we would have liked to gain traction with them very early on in the project.
>
> *Peter Perreiah, Director,*
> *PRHI*

Peter Perreiah, who had spent time working in industry, compares the people in industry with those in health care. (Most of this chapter is from an interview with him.)

> There are some major differences between health care and manufacturing. I really admire the passion and dedication that healthcare workers bring to the care of patients. No one can doubt that. What I have seen in the manufacturing industries is that the immediacy and grind of producing profitable results, month in and month out, brings a very intense focus on chang-

ing things for the better. Once you make some small changes in industry, you hang onto that gain. I think, too, the fierce global competition that a company like Alcoa in the aluminum business faces is absolutely clear to every person on the floor of that company. They are engaged in a battle to take cost out and reduce waste, so that every single year there is this overwhelming sense and urgency that things have to improve very, very rapidly. Nevertheless, I have great admiration for the innovation and the wonderful science that health care has produced.

I think part of the crisis (in healthcare) is fed by the way we educate and perhaps persuade ourselves that the problem necessarily has trade-offs. At Toyota, for example, they reject the idea that an improvement necessarily has to have a higher cost versus better patient outcomes versus a more responsive system. In Toyota the principle is that you go after all of those three goals simultaneously—better quality, lower cost, and more responsive systems. And you do that by understanding how problems arise from the system, so that by redesigning its smaller processes problem solving takes place at an ever-increasing pace.

Anyone who understands systems thinking realizes that small problems left unresolved may grow into larger problems. People who don't understand systems thinking tend to assign small importance to small problems. Consequently, they are less motivated, both personally and by the larger world, to focus their time and attention on smaller problems. Those who solve the larger, more complex problems tend to receive the accolades.

I'm not sure that everyone in health care is motivated to fix the small problems—the ones that add up to the large, complex and costly big problems. Not everyone is motivated because there are other distractions. For example, a research physician doesn't necessarily become famous for publishing papers on room cleaning, although that may be a very important issue throughout our hospitals. It is simply something not rewarded in the academic press. Let me explain.

124

I think the difference between industry and health care is that in manufacturing people focus on the parts. They see the small problems, whether it's making widgets or providing a simple service. They see them and are attacking them regularly. In health care we tend to roll the problems up into very complex ones. Problems often start out very small but quickly snowball into major complex problems, which require experts to resolve.

Moreover, it's often very difficult to understand the motivations for solving these problems. In a competitive industry, they have the month-in month-out incentive to actually produce a continually improving product. In health care, other motivations may intervene. Obviously, people do care about the patients. No one can cast doubt on that. But beyond that, the system doesn't necessarily always reward the resolution of those smaller problems. For example, many of the great minds in health care are working on very complex problems about which they can publish papers and make a name for themselves. It's very difficult to actually get a paper published on room cleaning, a problem which may impact many patients in terms of putting them at risk for contracting deadly pathogens.

Peter Perreiah, Director,
PRHI

CHANGING TIMES

Sometimes individual "workers" in a hospital believe they are truly helping a situation and giving best patient care. In the past being sure your patient had a wheelchair by hiding one in a bathroom might have been effective. In a larger, complex modern hospital it can create unintended and dangerous problems. Initiatives without knowledge of the system can backfire.

WHEELCHAIR STORY

Perreiah describes how the personnel at three VA facilities used systems thinking to solve a missing-wheelchairs problem. Anyone who wasn't yet a systems thinker when they first began resolving the scarcity of wheelchairs soon became one—by immersion.

125

We've been working on a very large project: to provide clean, appropriate wheelchairs to all our healthcare workers in their care of patients. This is a very large project because it involves the three different healthcare facilities here in the Pittsburgh area that serve veterans, each with different needs. In the long-term care facility, for example, patients sit in chairs for many hours; they have different needs from patients at the primary acute care facility who may only be visiting that facility and sitting in a chair for just a few hours.

The interesting thing about the wheelchair problem is that it is so large that people going about their work as a nurse, an escort, a clinical worker or a housekeeper—taking care of that rolling stock—only see a very small part of that large problem. Furthermore, they don't necessarily own the system of providing wheelchairs. So, they may not grasp or understand the larger problem, nor would they have the authority and the where-withal to actually begin to address the problems involved.

Nevertheless, to solve the problem, they needed the input of people who knew all the various parts of the system. Like the children's story about the blind men and the elephant, each of the healthcare personnel on the team knew one part of the whole problem but none of them could describe the whole problem or see a whole solution. Together, as each described his or her part of the wheelchair process, and as they sketched each part into one big picture on the board in front of them, the whole wheelchair system began to appear. Each one began to see the whole system and how the parts worked—or did not work—together. They were learning to think not only of their own small part, but also of the entire wheelchair system at the three VA hospitals. Studying wheelchairs led them into systems thinking.

This is an example of needing to gain support from the top, to get the various people in the system, who might contribute insights about the whole and the parts, to come together and describe, as it were, the total elephant and begin to redesign the entire system so that it works for everybody. This might involve, for example, getting together in one place escorts, people from nursing, housekeeping, security who are involved in preventing the loss of wheelchairs from the system, transportation, people who run wheelchairs back and forth between facilities, procurement who actually buy the wheelchairs, physical therapists who actually design wheelchairs and fit them to patient needs. This is a very complex problem. However, once we get people together who have insight about the various parts of the system, we can easily put it all together into a solution that works for everybody, saves a lot of time, and improves the care of patients. By a solution, I mean getting wheelchairs that not only support proper posture and comfort as well as make patients want to get up and stay active during the day, but also wheelchairs that are clean and don't transfer pathogens between users.

The idea then is to take the people who have the most insight about the way work is designed and focus on the many small problems and redesign the work so that these problems do not creep in and become very large problems.

ESTABLISHING THE CURRENT CONDITION OF THE PROBLEM

In addition to getting together the various groups who are involved in using wheelchairs, solving the problem as a systems thinker requires that everyone know the starting point, where the situation stands at present. Perreiah describes some of the issues they had to face:

We looked at a number of aspects of what we call the current condition. Just to enumerate a few of those: chairs were not always available to people who needed them. Often escorts would spend 10 to 20 minutes looking for a wheelchair. When they found one, it might not be appropriately outfitted. For example, it might not have leg rests that patients need to keep their feet up. It might not be sized right or might not have an oxygen tank holder on it, if the patient needed oxygen. There was a whole range of patient needs that were not necessarily being addressed. So the question was: how do we take the patient needs and redesign the system so that it can, first, recognize those needs, then respond to them without actually increasing the cost or the actual energy that goes into maintaining that system?

Here are some observations from a wheelchair escort for patients describing current conditions of the problem from his perspective.

> In the beginning, we had a problem finding wheelchairs, finding the right wheelchairs for the right patients, getting them to their appointments on time. It's been a problem for the nurses. They would get the patients ready and sometimes they needed to find things for a wheelchair, like leg rests, that they couldn't find or just weren't available.
>
> There are geriatric chairs. Some chairs recline, some don't. Some chairs have leg rests, and some don't. Some have oxygen tank holders, and some don't.
>
> There were enough chairs, but it was just hard to find them. On some floors people tried to hide them and they would disappear. When patients were being discharged, wheelchairs would be taken to the other hospital, and just getting them back was a problem.
>
> Sometimes our patients were late getting to their appointments, which backed other schedules up. It wasn't bad, but it was problem that needed to be addressed.
>
> *William Brown, Hospital Escort,*
> *VA Hospital, PRHI*

Wheelchairs are not simple machines and in many cases are not simply interchangeable. Therefore, the wheelchair problem is not just about the number of wheelchairs available. So, the solution involved more than the hospital staff that pushed patients around in wheelchairs.

PROBLEM SOLVING APPROACHES

Systems thinkers seldom follow traditional problem solving methods, Perreiah notes:

> We took a departure from the traditional way of problem solving. Traditionally, a hospital would have commissioned an expert team or committee who would study the problem at a high level for six to nine months and issue a report, which would then filter its way up to a manager who would make a decision

and put out a program. Our approach was a little bit different.

We said we don't want this committee of experts. What we would like is a team of people who actually work in using the wheelchairs and who work with patients and understand their needs. We got them together and said in the first week we actually want to begin to solve problems; that is, we want to form hypotheses about real problems that we know exist in different parts of the system. We also want to propose solutions and begin to test those solutions. Improving a system is an iterative process. We got to our final solution really on an ongoing way by repeatedly forming an hypothesis, testing it, and going back to the drawing board with improvements. With each iteration, we got finer and finer improvements, and kept getting better and better solutions.

We tested different styles of wheelchairs. We came up with new designs for outfitting wheelchairs. We went back and forth with different experts and users of those wheelchairs to see if they met the needs. In this way we actually arrived at the best design that we could come up with.

Peter Perreiah, Director,
PRHI

How Much Is Enough?

We're talking about approximately 500 wheelchairs among the three facilities. Obviously, there are a lot of them in the long-term care facility, which has 320 beds. At any point in time, many patients are in wheelchairs, so it's very hard for anyone to actually see all those 500 wheelchairs. As we got started, one of the interesting questions was: how many wheelchairs are in the hospital? We went around and asked people to guess. We actually had a contest. My supervisor at the initiative won the contest and she's not even actively involved in studying this problem. She took a wild guess and won.

The point here is that it's very hard for people to understand the system when they only see one part of it. What we found was that there are actually enough wheelchairs in the system;

however, they were not well-distributed and always available to people. For a lot of reasons. For example, we found it was very common for staff to hide and hoard wheelchairs. If in the past they had experienced that they could not find a wheelchair when they needed to take a patient, say, to an x-ray appointment, they would often pick up a wheelchair on their way into work and stash it in the bathroom in their unit, anticipating that they might not be able to find one during the shift.

You can imagine what happens if 12 people in each unit do that. We soon have 12 wheelchairs in the bathroom, the next day they do the same thing and we've got two-dozen wheelchairs hidden away. I'm exaggerating here but, in fact, many of the wheelchairs that could have served patients were being hidden in anticipation of a shortage, which in turn aggravated the shortage.

In an earlier time, individual nurses who hid wheelchairs in service of their personal patients might have been seen as clever, inventive, and committed to their patients. But from a systems viewpoint, nurses who sequestered wheelchairs for personal use were really aggravating the problem for the three hospitals. They weren't aware of the larger problem, so they solved their own need for a wheelchair, which in turn made it harder to solve the whole problem. Perreiah continues:

Our solution in this case was to address this question by a different approach: What is rational behavior when there is a shortage? We let people know about the problem, and that the ultimate solution to that problem was to put the resources, the wheelchairs, out in public and to have a fixed place in public where people knew they could go and get a wheelchair. We had to build some trust there. We had to actually make the wheelchairs available by putting together a system that insured, over time, if nurses or escorts went to that location there might only be two or three wheelchairs there, but they would always be available.

With that experience and the trust that was being built, they began to stop hiding and hoarding wheelchairs. The wheelchairs came out of the bathrooms and closets, and we soon had enough wheelchairs without purchasing a lot more and we freed up some space in those bathrooms.

The new wheelchair program was implemented throughout our three VA facilities because those facilities form a system. We exchange patients among them. Patients from the long-term care facility and from the psychiatric facility come to the acute care facility for clinic visits. For acute care we had to set up return loops to get the chairs back to the appropriate facilities because each place had different types of chairs. We did that by color-coding the wheelchairs according to facility and by identifying them with large numbers.

This proved to be a problem-solving solution in itself. If you go to, say, a long-term care facility and you see a blue wheelchair from the acute care facility, you know automatically that chair doesn't belong, and they need to put it back in the return loop so it will come back to its original hospital.

It took about year for us to work through all these solutions. It doesn't necessarily have to take that long to work through a normal problem. A lot of the wheelchair problem was an educational process. We were introducing a new set of principles. We were working on an extended problem that goes across different facilities and many different service lines. A typical problem like this at Toyota might take much less time. However, this was a learning experience and I'm sure that the next problem here at the VA, similar in nature and scope, will take far less time.

BENEFITS OF SYSTEMS THINKING

Even as they solved the problem of missing wheelchairs, they found ways to improve patient care.

Some of the benefits of the new wheelchair program are very direct. They go right to the patients in terms of comfort. They can sit in a chair for a long period of time. For example, at our long term care facility, we now have seat cushions on all the chairs. The back heights were designed high enough to accommodate the seat cushions. Things like this are very important in improving the health of those patients. They want to get out of bed. Getting patients out of bed is important to prevent urinary tract infections and pneumonias in the long term. It's also very important to keep patients active to reduce the incidence of ulcers that occur because of prolonged motionlessness in a bed.

Obviously, the chairs are cleaned, reducing the infection risk.

There are other benefits to the system, too. It reduces the frustration for the healthcare worker. The wheelchair system really went from being an emblem of how things can't work at the VA to an emblem of how things can work if we all pull together, and we agreed to set up and to follow these principles. So it was a very positive experience.

REDUCING WASTE

One of the many benefits of systems thinking is that it often helps reduce waste—sometimes it is waste that was never considered waste before—by continually improving processes within the system.

We put in some security measures. For example, on each wheelchair we put a phone number that could be called 7 days a week, 24 hours a day if someone were to find a wheelchair off site.

The first month we put phone numbers on we got 40 chairs back—40 chairs returned to the VA that in the past would have been dead losses. The VA would have to purchase new chairs for the ones that got lost. There are many benefits, both economic and psychologically, in terms of patient care.

A lot of wasted time was also saved. It's hard to always add up every minute that's saved. You know there's direct time that's saved because an escort doesn't have to go searching for a wheelchair that a nurse has hidden. All wheelchairs are outfitted with the legs and an oxygen tank holder, so that an escort can grab that wheelchair, put the patient in it, and take them off to their appointment.

But there are other kinds of lost minutes in time that you don't ordinarily notice. For example, a person who has found a wheelchair that's, say, contaminated by a former user has to stop and clean it up. That is an issue of wasted time. We now have a very tight regularly scheduled cleaning of the wheelchairs. Moreover, we have materials readily available so that people can spot clean a dirty chair. All these things save time.

We also have designed a system to re-circulate all our chairs, so that people don't spend time rearranging extra chairs at different facilities or chairs that haven't been returned yet.

Obviously, having wheelchairs available when you need them, if you're a healthcare worker, is very important. It's a source of frustration if you don't have a wheelchair to serve your patient immediately and have to stop your routine and hunt for one. So, it's a big boost to know that the hospital is supporting you with the appropriate equipment to do your work.

Peter Perreiah, Director,
PRHI

Now, we have assigned wheelchair places. We clean our wheelchairs after every use. We have different areas where wheelchairs are stocked, so if we run out of chairs on the floor we have a place to get them in a timely manner. We've got new wheelchairs. A lot of wheelchairs now have legs on them so we're not hunting for parts. They all have oxygen tank holders. All the tanks have regulators on them now, so we're not going from floor to floor looking for regulators, which was also time consuming.

Patients are coming here from different units. You never know who's been sitting in what and who has what disease, so it's my responsibility on my floor to keep the wheelchairs I stock clean. I clean them all. Wheelchairs are kept the same way on any other floor.

Today, I have a lot more responsibility, which is good, because I'm not standing around with nothing to do when there's nobody to escort. I'm stocking the cupboards, making sure the nurses have their supplies, cleaning my wheelchairs, cleaning my stretchers, making sure we've got supplies for what the nurses need.

It's a wonderful environment here. All the nurses are great. Everybody's nice. Everybody's friendly. The patients are wonderful. And as long as we're making them happy, that's all that matters.

William Brown, Hospital Escort,
VA Hospital, PRHI

Nurses Handoff Report Story

PRHI's director tells another story of nurses who learned how to apply systems thinking to a bothersome and time-consuming, but essential, process in their work.

One of our first tasks when we began the implementation of systems thinking for nurses in our existing system here was to understand the stability of that system. We found, for example, that the nurses were often in a hurry. They were pressed for time. So we asked them the simple question: How can we save you time?

One of the things we found was that they were spending a considerable amount of time actually doing a hand-off to their replacements, the nurses coming in on the next shift.

Peter Perreiah, Director,
PRHI

It is very important for the new shift nurses to know what happened to each of their patients during the previous eight hours and what the current condition of each patient is. Before the new nurses take charge of the unit, the nurse leaving the unit must prepare a written report on each patient. Using this handoff report, the departing nurse reviews the status of each patient with the nurse coming on the unit for the next shift. Each nurse had her own way of creating and delivering this report. Perreiah continues:

Before one shift left for the day, they would spend considerable time preparing a hand-off report for each patient. When we first started studying the hand-off process, it often involved various forms—written documents, things recorded on a computer, a taped report on the patient, as well as facts that were related verbally nurse-to-nurse. We looked at that whole process and

134

worked with the nurses to find out the essential information they needed to do their hand-off.

Initially, our goal was saving them some time. As we got into it with them, we found out this was a complex problem. We asked the nurses to break this problem down into simple parts and to look at the different modes of communication they had been using, and the actual item-by-item content of information that was being handed off to the next shift. When looked at in this way, they found out there were actually a number of simple problems. We worked at them, one by one.

Almost all problems in health care that seem to create minor crises and much waste arise from the failure to see how the parts are connected to the whole and how, once people see the whole system, they can break down the problem's solution into smaller, more easily solvable parts. In the nurses' hand-off problem, one of the smaller problems was describing a patient's diagnosis clearly and succinctly. It turned out there were about forty such diagnoses to describe.

Some nurses, for example, took diagnoses home, pulled out their old nursing notebooks, and wrote down the key elements that they needed to report when a certain patient had that diagnosis. Now, there are over 40 diagnoses that come through our inpatient surgery floor, so as a whole, identifying key elements for each diagnosis is a very challenging problem for any individual nurse to solve. As a team though, our nurses were very effective in delineating the important facts that needed to be shared in hand-offs on each of these diagnoses.

And they didn't stop there. They took this detailed knowledge, which had now been simplified into checklists, and designed it into a pattern for doing an overall report. Today, the hand-off report that everyone uses starts with a general description of the patient, follows with a general assessment, drops to a specific assessment, and concludes with some overall description of patient response and behavior.

In other words, the nurses had developed a way of standardizing all hand-off reports, so that in every report information was presented in the same order, reducing confusion and time wasted.

This was initially done in an informal way using checklists. Next, the checklist was standardized onto a laminated sheet, which is still in use. We traced its effectiveness and after several months some improvement ideas came in about putting the hand-off into the computer to save some further time. We aren't quite finished implementing the hand-off process, but we have a lot of insight as to how to build that computer interface. We've actually done some point-and-click work.

So, the improvement began by translating their original good thinking onto check sheets that evolved into a laminated flow sheet that is now in the computer available for their use, if they choose to use it.

Overall, we've seen some dramatic benefits. Whereas nurses used to spend 45 to 60 minutes doing a shift change, they now spend 20 to 30 minutes. But beyond the timesaving, more importantly, all the nurses feel that they now give a better quality report. They give more complete and clearly patterned information, so that it's very easy to recognize whenever something is missing.

STANDARDIZATION

In developing a more effective and efficient hand-off reporting system, the nurses had done it themselves, without calling in experts to solve their problems for them. They had taken an approach similar to one used in manufacturing, using tools they had learned from Toyota. Perreiah continues:

In manufacturing, facing a small problem, people are much more ready to pick up a hammer or a set of pliers to come up with a solution themselves. In health care, many of the systems are brought in from the outside. The expert electronic devices we have now are brought in from the outside and no doubt they work very well for what they do. But that takes away the experience of resolving very small problems in a sort of homespun way. When you lose that experience, you lose the ability to solve more sophisticated problems. Toyota has a system that's evolved some very elegant and sophisticated solutions, for example, about planning and scheduling. They've found

136

solutions over the course of 50 years, starting with very simple approaches.

Many of the scheduling problems that we see in an operating room or in different hospital units are analogous to those in manufacturing. But what we haven't seen is this evolution of real-time problem solving on the hospital floor. In health care, the solutions that we have seen often come in from outside, from technical experts or scheduling experts who have created software systems to resolve certain problems. This doesn't empower people to solve their own problems on the floor.

These nurses, however, had been empowered to solve their own problem in real time, step-by-step and stage-by-stage, continually improving the process.

Learning the Toyota system is empowering hospital personnel with a set of skills and with the okay from management to do experiments. They learned to do them in a way that limits risk to the organization, but in a way that enriches their experience so they have further insight to take those same skills and go further. After solving problem A, they go on to solve problems B, C and D, which may be more complicated.

Furthermore, they built every improvement into the process itself, so that the improvements they made would be permanent.

A common question is asked. Is this improvement sustainable? Will they keep using what they have learned? Will it go on after I leave as a teacher or after the team leaders that we've trained may be transferred? That is a very good question. Toyota's system, like all other systems, needs to be sustained. Systems are sustained through training of individuals, but importantly they're also sustained in the way procedures and processes are set up.

A continually improving organization should have a structure that reinforces the problem-solving skills with each challenge that people encounter. This reinforces a problem-solving organization. Standardized work—standardizing the way people do their tasks, following a sequence of steps, and continually reflecting on that work—is very important for sustaining this work. We standardize work to the one best way and then people experiment from there, seeking further improvements. They begin to think, "Well maybe it doesn't make sense. It's common sense not to do it a different way because it will be harder, it will be less safe. It might produce an outcome that is not as favorable."

One of the best ways to make sure this continual improvement is sustainable is to actually design it into the work *so it doesn't make sense to do it any other way.* This can take the form of the actual listing of tasks that people do. It can be embedded in the environment, in the artifacts that people work with, the way machines are designed, and the way rooms are laid out. Or it may be embedded in the relationships that they build with suppliers or customers or their services. Once those are standardized and set up in an agreed upon manner, it becomes common sense to do it the one way and not to do it the other way.

Peter Perreiah, Director,
PRHI

Another part of sustainability and standardization is data feedback to the process users so they can easily see if there is a fall-off in performance.

The nurses, doctors and healthcare staff didn't one day just start learning systems thinking, seeing with new eyes, understanding processes and beginning to practice continual improvement. Their leaders had to understand it first and give up many of their old practices and ideas. They talk about it in the next chapter.

SOME THINGS TO REMEMBER FROM THIS CHAPTER

✓ Just doing your best doesn't work in complex organizations.

✓ People must understand the system and its often hidden interactions and connections between people and the parts.

✓ Seeing the whole system is not easy because it is different from our habitual, individualistic approach to thinking and working.

✓ Solving healthcare problems does not have to have trade-offs, e.g., patient safety does not have to mean higher costs.

✓ Small problems—dirty floors, missing rubber gloves—can quickly lead to big problems.

✓ An effective way to learn systems thinking is for the frontline team to work together to observe, describe and propose solutions to a problem.

✓ Fixing one problem can lead to many unexpected solutions, e.g., making wheelchairs readily available had many benefits: better chairs, reduced costs, clean chairs, personnel who understood systems thinking, etc.

CHAPTER 12

WHAT OUR LEADERSHIP LEARNED

Twenty-five years ago...a group of us in a hospital would sit around in a room and we would design the health delivery system for that facility. We would decide what the customers wanted and what they would get out of it. They got waiting rooms with long waits and magazines that were two- or three-years old. They got hospitals where you walk in; you're scared to death because you don't know which way to turn, and you don't know where to go. You got bad food and bad attitudes, because we had a certain sense of arrogance. We knew better than the people out there what they should get and what they needed when they came in.

Kevin Kast, President,
SSM St. Joseph's Health Center

If an organization and its staff are to become systems thinkers, the leadership must first change its role and function. Hierarchy essentially disappears and leadership moves horizontally, alongside all other functions in the organization, primarily as holder and committed promoter of the new corporate vision.

Paul O'Neill led the hospital improvement program in Pittsburgh. Sister Mary Jean Ryan led it in St. Louis. He is a former government bureaucrat, who became a successful CEO of Alcoa and Secretary of the Treasury; she is a nurse and a nun. It is difficult to think of two people who come from more different backgrounds, yet they both reached exactly the same realization. Each hospital is a system, not merely a collection of departments. To heal a hospital requires three things. First, leadership; it is the role of the leader to establish goals that everyone can relate to. Second, the aim of any healthcare system must be continually improving patient care. PRHI called it "perfect patient care." SSM called it "exceptional patient care" aiming for the 99th percentile. Third, a leader—and as many others as possible—needs to be a systems thinker.

DEVELOPING A SYSTEMS THINKING LEADER

W. Edwards Deming formulated "Fourteen Points" that characterize his quality management method. They are directed to leaders, managers, and supervisors who are responsible for creating and maintaining an organizational system designed for continual improvement of employees, goods and services. The Fourteen Points are a radical approach to organizational change compared to traditional management.

Taken together they allow leaders to create an organization in which everyone—workers and managers—can experience joy in work as they produce increasingly effective and efficient goods and services. In hospitals that would be better and safer patient care.

THE FOURTEEN POINTS

1. Create constancy of purpose toward improvement of product and service
2. Adopt the new philosophy.
3. Cease dependence on inspection to achieve quality.
4. End the practice of awarding business on the basis of price tag.
5. Improve constantly and forever the system of production and service.
6. Institute training on the job.
7. Institute leadership.
8. Drive out fear so everyone may work effectively.
9. Break down barriers between departments.
10. Eliminate slogans, exhortations and targets for the work force.
11.a Eliminate work standards (quotas).
11.b Eliminate management by objective.
12. Remove barriers that rob (employees) of their pride of workmanship.
13. Institute a vigorous program of education and self-improvement.
14. Put everyone in the (organization) to work to accomplish the transformation.

Deming formulated the Fourteen Points in the late 1970s as he observed the differences between Japanese electronic and automobile manufacturers, such as Toyota, and their US competitors. They became the basis of his books and lectures.

He said another way of expressing the Fourteen Points was as a System of Profound Knowledge:

1) An appreciation for a system.
2) An understanding that there is variation in all things, requiring an appreciation for statistical knowledge and decision-making based on fact.
3) An understanding of how people learn.
4) An understanding of what motivates people and how they behave in organizations.

He said a manager does not have to be an expert in any of these fields, but must be aware of these theories and how their interaction can help an organization be greater than the sum of its parts.

HISTORIC VIEWPOINT

Russell Ackoff approaches systems thinking and the leadership of modern organizations from a historical point of view. In the 19th Century, organizations or corporations were viewed as machines, which operated for the benefit of the owner. The workers were viewed as interchangeable parts.

As corporations grew bigger early in the 20th Century, they were viewed as biological systems with various and different parts working for the aim of the business. Employees had different jobs and worked together for the benefit of the owners or stockholders and to maintain the lifestyle of management. The leader of the biological corporation was called "the head."

The parts or people in the system, just like the parts of the human body, were seen as having no separate or personal agendas. (Your liver only works to maintain your body.)

By the middle of World War II, workers for large organizations were working not just for money, but to win the war. Many were women and needed childcare and other considerations. These employees or "parts" were interested in the aim of the organization but also had separate, personal aims. Such organizations, in which the departments and employees have their own agendas as well as the company aim form a new kind of system called a complex social organization. According to Dr. Ackoff, managing these contemporary organizations requires new and continually improving leadership skills—even more so in a rapidly changing world. A hospital is a complex social system.

INSTITUTE LEADERSHIP

By including Point 7, Institute leadership, it is clear that Deming believes that systems-thinking leadership is absent in most organizations, so he requires that it be *instituted*. Under this point, he directs his advice to line managers and supervisors. "The job of a supervisor is not to tell people what to do or punish them, but to lead. Leading consists of helping people do a better job and of learning by objective methods who is in need of individual help."

Deming was very fond of repeating the adage, "Leadership cannot be delegated." He was also fond of saying, "The world would be a better place if people who do their best would stay at home in bed." He would go on to explain that best efforts are not enough, people need systems knowledge.

Managing a complete conversion to systems thinking in an organization as complex and multi-layered as a hospital presents a mammoth task, because it requires orchestrating a complete change of mind, heart and behavior for almost every person in the organization—a change of culture.

How does a leader formulate an aim or purpose—a vision for the whole organization—to which everyone in the organization will willingly and readily commit? Such an aim or vision must be, at the same time, compelling, inspiring, un-rejectable, irresistible, and something everyone can understand and relate to.

How does a leader maintain his enthusiasm for the vision, over time and throughout the organization? It requires a leader's complete dedication and energy, and it must become the central, most important purpose of his or her leadership activity. The leader must have a game plan for success, and must oversee and nurture the transformation each day and every day for every employee.

The leadership at PRHI and SSM Health Care quickly discovered that most of the traditional leadership qualities they had inherited from previous generations of leaders would not effect such a transformation and did not fit within a systems thinking mentality.

In this chapter, we hear how various leaders, managers, and supervisors discovered that they had to completely rethink what it meant to truly lead or manage people in a large system. They had a lot of learning to absorb and often stumbled in trying to translate it into appropriate behavior.

We look at the leadership in each healthcare system in turn.

LEADERSHIP AT SSM HEALTH CARE

SSM Health Care owns, operates, and manages 22 facilities, including 20 acute care hospitals in four states. CEO, Sister Mary Jean Ryan, its senior vice president, William P. Thompson, and others describe how they introduced a program of Continual Quality Improvement (CQI) and what leadership had to do at SSM Health Care. Sister describes how it was when leaders were expected to be in total control of everything and could step into any crisis, as if they were the Lone Ranger or Mighty Mouse, to save the day.

> Our cultures have spawned a whole lot of aberrations in terms of behaviors, but one of our early consultants talked about Mighty Mouse and the Lone Ranger. Everybody knew what they were talking about. The Lone Ranger is somebody who absolutely has to make decisions by himself or herself. That doesn't work in a culture where we are focusing on teamwork. You cannot be a Lone Ranger in that instance. To make decisions alone without conferring with anybody else is just a deadly way of operating.
>
> I remember when I've done this myself. In my earlier days as a department head or supervisor, somebody would come to me with a problem that had been going on for a few days and they'd say, "What do you want us to do?" and I'd say, "Well, do this, this and this." That's Mighty Mouse going in to save the day.
>
> With CQI I learned to say to people, "Look, that's your problem. You know I'll help you in any way that I can but it's going to be your problem to solve because you know more about that

than I do." But making that shift from the old language was hard for me. When someone came to me with a problem asking what he or she should do, for me to say "I don't know" was one of the hardest things to get over. And yet if we leaders don't get over that, we continue making bad decisions and we don't develop people to the fullest extent of their capacity. In my mind, the development of other people is such a critical aspect of all of this. And, you know, neither the Lone Ranger nor Mighty Mouse lend themselves to that.

I think that medical schools are probably notorious for turning out Lone Rangers and Mighty Mouses...though more and more schools are beginning to recognize that when these people get out into actual practice they're going to have to be working with other people.

Sister Mary Jean Ryan, FSM, RN, President & CEO,
SSM Health Care

Sister took a view which was pretty radical, particularly in the late 80s, that there's a lot more we could be doing and you can't blame it on Medicare reimbursement or managed care or other problems. She said that, while all of the real issues and challenges like that exist in health care, we could at the same time be improving care. And her mindset is just very different.

William Schoenhard, Executive VP & COO,
SSM Health Care

People in leadership had to give up the thought of acting like a Lone Ranger or a Mighty Mouse in order to move into systems thinking and continual quality improvement. Leadership needed to be dispersed throughout the organization. Every employee needed to learn to think of the good of the whole system, not just of their corner of the hospital.

It is not easy to shift mindsets.

We introduced the plan that we were going to adopt the principles of continual quality improvement, the purpose of which was to change the culture of this organization. It was not necessary to get better but *to create a culture committed to getting better,* which we thought was really the foundation of what we had to do.

William P. Thompson, Senior Vice President,
Strategic Development, SSM Health Care

And without executive leadership absolutely committed to quality over the long haul, you're not going to be able to do it.

Paul Convery, MD, Chief Medical Officer
SSM Health Care/St. Louis

The other important piece is that within any organization the senior leadership including the CEO needs to be very support-ive of that work.... Sister Mary Jean is the change agent in this organization. When Sister Mary Jean became convinced that CQI was the approach we wanted to take and that it described the culture we were trying to create in this organization, her unwavering commitment to it has been absolutely essential for the progress of this organization. There have been multiple oc-casions over the last 13 years when people have gone to Sister Mary Jean and said, "Sister, we can't afford to do this. We can-not take the time out of our busy schedules to do CQI. We can't find a time to make improvement."

William P. Thompson, Senior Vice President,
Strategic Development, SSM Health Care

If I get really convinced about something, I can be pretty con-vincing. I did not want to use my position to do that. I wanted everybody to be able to say, "Yes, we agree with you, not be-cause you're the boss but because we think it's the right thing to do." That's really the way we came to CQI.

Sister Mary Jean Ryan, FSM, RN, President & CEO,
SSM Health Care

She's an extremely driving force. She is the force behind the Malcolm Baldrige Award, behind our CQI, behind the excellence in response; she's an extremely stimulating person that you want to accomplish these things for.

Tim Thompson, DO, Emergency Room Director
SSM St Joseph's Hospital West

First, we had to redefine the role of management. At one point in time we looked at management as a hierarchical position. You started out as a worker, and then you were promoted to management.

Over the past few years, we've come to recognize that management isn't a hierarchy; it's simply a different function in the system. So, you have employees here and you have management here, and they work together to accomplish a goal and objective.

The role of management is also different. It goes from being a boss to being a mentor and facilitator and supporter. That was a significant change for us, and we're still working through that with many of our middle management and upper management.

William P. Thompson, Senior Vice President,
Strategic Development, SSM Health Care

A lot of people are banging on the doors to learn more about trust since we won the Baldrige Award. The resistance can come from leadership. It can come sometimes from ignorance and lack of awareness of thinking this way. In some cases the clinicians and the staff themselves may resist that freedom. Maybe I'm not sure I can report a near miss and not be punished. It takes a long time to move from what traditionally in hospitals has been a hierarchical command and control to management that really invites innovation, creativity and freedom.

William Schoenhard, Executive VP & COO,
SSM Health Care

What a systems approach has allowed us to do from this level is articulate some very explicit goals and expectations, starting with our mission statement. "Through our exceptional health care services we reveal the healing presence of God."

We have created a series of values around stewardship, justice, respect, and quality. That message has been clearly articulated and communicated. We have identified certain characteristics of exceptional health care because we realize not everyone understood what exceptional healthcare services meant. So, we went through an exercise and, in the end, we said, "For us, exceptional health care means exceptional clinical outcomes, exception satisfaction of our employees, our patients, and our physicians and exceptional financial results." We recognize that exceptional health care includes all of those components.

William P. Thompson, Senior Vice President,
Strategic Development, SSM Health Care

Sister's a very practical person. She's very much sort of nuts and bolts, back to basics, and fundamental, always reminding us: what is our purpose, what is our mission? What is our vision? That constant emphasis and singular focus has led us on this path to continued improvement. She doesn't espouse the fad of the month or the fad of the week, but it's constancy of purpose. That has been very characteristic of her leadership style.

Paula Friedman, Vice President, Systems Improvement,
SSM Health Care

Sister can take mission/vision across an organization and deploy it consistently, so that you see it as a common thread in everything that you do. It's not improvements in singular areas, but it's looking at it across the whole of an organization.

Paula Friedman, Vice President, Systems Improvement,
SSM Health Care

Sister is very clear about what she wants. Her expectations do not change and that's very helpful for those of us within our organization. Her strategy is very patient-focused. She's a nurse and it's obvious that patients are very important to her and that improvement needs to occur every day.

Eunice Halverson, Corporate Vice President
Quality Resource Center, SSM Health Care

Sister Mary Jean, unlike any other health care CEO in the United States, really consistently calls our system to continuous improvement. I don't know of any other CEO over this period of time since 1989 that has had the constancy of purpose and the personal commitment to challenge all of us to learn more about the process of care and the continuance of improvement. I've seen CEOs in health care get excited about this, try it and then get disillusioned and move on to the next management fad of the month. To her credit, she never wavered from this commitment and believed, even at a time when many people were cynical and questioning, that this would ultimately improve the quality of care to patients. She often gives everyone throughout our system credit for winning the Baldrige Award, but it would not have occurred without her leadership.

We are focused on a much broader array of measurements in clinical outcomes and satisfaction that were never really thought of in a systematic way in 1989. And all of this is translated to improved market share, profitability and growth of this system than was certainly the case in 1989.

William Schoenhard, Executive VP & COO,
SSM Health Care

LEADERSHIP AT THE PITTSBURGH REGIONAL HEALTHCARE INITIATIVE (PRHI)

PRHI, you may recall, involves 41 different affiliates, including not only competing hospitals and various other healthcare facilities, but local employers and some health insurance companies. Karen Wolk Feinstein was the founder of PRHI and Paul O'Neill was its first CEO.

For me, the foundation of how to think about things begins with a belief that the world can be an ever better place for everyone. There are conditions that are preconditions to establish that possibility. One of those preconditions is leadership.

Let me define for you what I mean by leadership. I don't mean cheerleading. What I mean is leadership in every kind of organization—public, private, non-profit—has an essential role: to create the conditions in an organization so that all the human beings in it can say yes, without delay, to three questions every day. The three questions are these:

- Are you treated with dignity and respect every day by everyone you encounter?

- Are you being given what you need including training and tools and whatever is necessary for you to make a contribution that gives meaning to your life?

- Did someone notice you did it?

And I think those are kind of preconditions for an organization to become excellent.

Paul O'Neill, former U.S. Treasury Secretary,
Former CEO, PRHI

THREE IMPORTANT QUESTIONS

O'Neill's three questions above should be underlined as they form the basis of his management philosophy. To the degree they are fulfilled, they create a culture of care and meaningfulness throughout an organization. With such a culture in place, a leader can get buy-in from employees, suppliers, and customers for most goals he proposes.

Now, with an understanding that those are preconditions, it's the role of the leader to establish goals that everyone can relate to. Again, this is not about making more money or some of the things many leaders in a private enterprise would say they're here to make. Great organizations respond to goals that are important in life or for other people. For example, a really inspiring goal I found in my career in both public and private sector is to say to people, "One of the things that we should do in our organization is create the conditions so that no one is ever hurt at work." No one can argue that that's not a valuable goal. It's also a kind of a goal that has an inspirational quality to it.

Once you've established a worthy goal that binds people together, then you need some tools to actually achieve your goal. And those tools include giving people eyes that can see. After you've established a worthy goal like "No one gets hurt at work," you need to give people tools so that they can move in a conscious way toward the achievement of the goal.

Paul O'Neill, former U.S. Treasury Secretary,
Former CEO, PRHI

A hospital is not a factory. It is hard to change things overnight. And when you are fitting a change process into a very complex environment like a hospital, you have to do this very carefully with people who really know the culture and the workings of the hospital. It's very hard to impose a framework, even though it's worked exquisitely well in other settings, on a hospital.

Karen Wolk Feinstein, Chair & Founder, PRHI,
President, Jewish Healthcare Foundation

We are trying to do our homework in this area because we understand that in health care everything else has been tried. The "do less" has been tried, the "paying less" has been tried. There is nothing left than "doing better." And to do better is applying continuous improvement and the quality movement to health care as a process.

Alberto Colombi, MD, Chief Medical Officer,
PPG Industries

You won't get very far with continual process improvement without the complete support of the leadership, because in that transformation you're really going against the undertow of all the inertia and current ways of doing work. This Toyota Production System asks you to set that aside for a while and become acquainted with a direction and strategy for the design of work that is completely different than the way we see things today.

David Sharbaugh, Director of Quality Improvement,
PRHI

151

As a leader of a team involved in a quality process, it's like anything else, you lead from the front. If you don't believe that having a disciplined approach to quality or that understanding the specifics are important, if you don't believe that having a game plan that is detailed and well understood by the entire team is critical to the success of that team—if you don't believe those things, your team won't pick up and be effective. So, first of all, you've got to be committed. You've got to believe and you've got to be committed to it.

Raymond LeBoeuf, CEO,
PPG Industries

OTHER LEADERS

Others in leadership positions come from different perspectives. A nurse sees leadership from the front lines. The CEO of PPG Industries volunteers his time at PRHI because his agenda is to reduce premiums his company has to pay healthcare insurers by making hospitals in his area more effective and efficient. And a president of a hospital in PRHI reluctantly finds her way into the new world by following the crowd.

I think the first way is to lead by example. I have not asked any of my leadership staff to go out and participate in these improvement activities without me doing it first.

Tami Merryman, RN, Vice President, Patient Care Services,
Shadyside Hospital, PRHI

As a leader, you've got to be willing to be measured and held accountable for your part of the process. It isn't the rest of the team that's being measured or the rest of the process that's being measured. It's the entire process, and that includes the leadership. So, I think it's very important that a leader understand what the discipline that the team is being asked to adopt is all about, and be committed to it and be willing to be measured by it.

Raymond LeBoeuf, CEO,
PPG Industries

I didn't believe it at first and I really only started to go to the meetings and participate because everyone in the region was going and participating. It was actually the application of some of these tools and techniques and some things that occurred here at Allegheny General Hospital in the last 8 to 12 months that made me a believer. I actually saw things improve—outcomes improving and doing what is right for the patient. So, I saw results and that's what proved it to me.

Connie Cibrone, President & CEO,
Allegheny General Hospital, PRHI

SOME THINGS TO REMEMBER FROM THIS CHAPTER

✓ Leaders create the vision.

✓ Hierarchy in the traditional sense essentially disappears.

✓ Leaders change from boss to mentor, facilitator and supporter.

✓ Leaders work alongside other staff primarily as stakeholders and promoters of the corporate vision.

✓ Leaders become continual learners and involve everyone in the transformation.

✓ Leaders lead change to a culture of dignity, respect and acknowledgement.

✓ Leaders insure that everyone has the proper tools and training.

PART III:

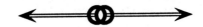

The Path of Improvement

CHAPTER 13

GOING FOR THE
THEORETICAL LIMIT

Our goal of perfect patient care means that, for example, every person who has diabetes or depression should get that effective care that's already been proven by research—that the care will be as perfect as it can be based on what is accepted medical knowledge at the time.

Tania Lyon, Ph.D., Chronic Care Coordinator,
PRHI

DEFECT-FREE HEALTH CARE

An insistence on continual improvement of all processes and systems has always been the cornerstone of organizational transformation as practiced by Toyota and others who follow the systems-thinking-based Deming teachings.

This continual-improvement approach requires that the shared aim or purpose for unifying and inspiring an entire organization be a larger vision, one that can never be fully attained.

For example, Fujio Cho, President of Toyota, wrote in The Toyota Way document, 2001, "Since Toyota's founding we have adhered to the core-principle of contributing to society through the practice of manufacturing high-quality products and services." Yet the same defect-free automobile is not enough to continue to satisfy and delight Toyota owners. Why? Because each year new technical advances are being made which need to be incorporated into their vehicles, and each year customer expectations increase and wish lists for their vehicles grow longer. Who would have thought a decade ago that customers would expect CD players, television sets, global positioning systems and the like to be standard equipment or hybrid cars powered by electricity as well as gasoline engines?

156

However, health care is a different world. No U.S. healthcare facilities provide defect-free treatment, which is why hospitals themselves are in need of healing. The sober fact is that somewhere near 100,000 patients die unnecessarily each year from hospital-acquired infections. And fourteen times that number acquire those infections but manage to survive, at great expense, suffering and frequently permanent disability. This number of fatal or nearly fatal infections includes neither outright medical and surgical mistakes nor incorrect or improper medications delivered. It does not include those hundreds, if not thousands, of "near misses" luckily caught each day by an observant nurse moments before administering a wrong medication to a patient.

In the following pages, people engaged in the systems-thinking transformation of their hospitals use a number of expressions to capture the same driving purpose. "Striving for perfect patient care," "going for the theoretical limit," and "reaching for the ideal" are three of these expression that convey a similar meaning. These are lofty positive aims, high above the zero line on a performance graph.

However, today's hospitals generate many unnecessary mistakes, infections and deaths. From this point of view, they are just starting their upward climb from the negative side—below zero—of the performance graph. In order to get their negative scores *up to zero*—odd as that must sound—they first need to achieve defect-free service. Striving for defect-free outcomes has been the primary work, so far, of hospitals healing themselves. Just getting to defect-free service is a major accomplishment and can take years.

Yet despite mistakes, infections and unnecessary deaths, hospitals are still saving the lives of many more people than they could have helped a few years ago. This is why approaching continual improvement can sound more complicated than it is practice.

Toyota has been producing defect-free automobiles for decades. They assume a defect-free product as their starting point for continual improvement and customer satisfaction. Every improvement they achieve now is on the positive side of the graph.

Even though this back-to-zero drive among the healthcare systems we studied has been a monumental achievement, when they finally accomplish it, they will only be crossing the zero threshold and entering the positive side of the graph. They will have miles and miles to go yet to reach the ideal, the theoretical limit, of "perfect patient care."

The sad fact is that hospitals wanting to improve are starting out with a defect-laden healthcare delivery system. And the errors and mistakes mean prolonged sickness or even death for their customers, their patients, as well as huge costs—all unnecessary.

Remember Dr. Steven J. Spear in the *Harvard Business Review* predicts that if Toyota principles were applied in every American hospital and medical errors were reduced by 90 percent, 87,700 patients would avoid injury, 39,600 to 88,200 lives would be saved and $15.3 billion to $26.1 billion would be saved annually.

Since patient health and safety was the main concern at PRHI and SSM, their leadership could not be content with mere incremental improvements in reducing hospital mistakes. The improvements had to be radical and fast. They felt it was not enough for them to say, "Let's reduce hospital-aquired infections by 10 percent."

PRHI and SSM Health Care chose to set their goals at zero deaths from hospital-acquired infections, zero medication errors, zero medical mistakes. Although they realized they might not ever reach zero infections, errors or mistakes, they could not, morally or ethically, set their sights on anything less. After all, they realized, even if they accomplished this impossible goal, all they could claim is that they were now offering the baseline of good health care—defect-free products and services—a defect-free baseline Toyota had been providing in its automobiles for decades.

Nonetheless, these hospital systems seeking such safety perfection in healthcare as their goal was revolutionary. It was dramatically different from the old "zero defects" slogan of manufacturing in the 1980s and 90s, which was an exhortation without a method to achieve it—similar to "Do It Right the First Time!" heard also in the 1980s. Again, no method for doing it was offered.

Even though neither PRHI nor SSM Health Care has yet to achieve totally defect-free health care delivery, they have made dramatic improvement. They are healing their healthcare facilities because they never stop trying to get better. More improvement is always possible.

THE "THEORETICAL LIMIT" CONCEPT

Paul O'Neill derived the theoretical limit concept while he was CEO of Alcoa. Soon after he arrived there, he called for a commitment to perfect safety for all Alcoa employees as well as customers or suppliers on Alcoa property. He called for zero accidents and zero safety incidents throughout Alcoa's hundreds of plants and offices in countries around the globe.

O'Neill tells the story of meeting the company safety director for the first time and telling him that it was unacceptable that Alcoa's present safety record was the "best in our industry." To the startled director, O'Neill said, "From today onward our objective is perfect safety for all people who have anything to do with Alcoa."

Employees at Alcoa didn't immediately sign up for perfect safety. They were so used to accidents happening that they refused to believe it was possible. So, O'Neill began making visits to different plants "to make sure that everybody understood that perfect safety was my first objective."

To management, he said, "People who work at Alcoa should never be hurt. If you identify something that can be done to make your plant safer, you should go do it immediately. You should not put it in next year's budget and hope that in the meantime no one will get hurt. Whatever promotes total safety is always in the budget."

To the hourly workers, "If management doesn't follow up on what I just said to them, here's my home phone number. Call me." Management couldn't believe he would give them his home phone number, but he did. He received only a few phone calls from workers telling him that good safety ideas were being rejected. As soon as managers realized O'Neill was serious and would take swift action, phone calls were no longer necessary.

Although statisticians and quality experts told O'Neill what he wanted to accomplish in such a short time was impossible, he would stand up at employee meetings and ask, "Please raise your hand if you would be willing to be an Alcoa accident victim this year." When no hands went up, everyone realized that everyone else—every single person in the company—desired this goal of perfect safety and were willing to strive for it. That's when he knew he had their shared commitment to pursue this goal to its theoretical limit.

Of course, a "theoretical limit" goal is precisely that, a limit that can be attained only in theory. But, as O'Neill said, it was the first goal that deserved striving for. In less than eight years, Alcoa became the safest company in the world to work for, despite the fact that employees work with massive machines, heavy equipment, and molten aluminum all day long. And importantly, profits increased dramatically as people learned to work together better.

In his pursuit of the theoretical limit, O'Neill discovered that benchmarking was really a bad idea. "If you follow a benchmarking approach," he said, "you're supposed to find the best there is and try to be like that. If we at Alcoa had stopped after matching Dupont's safety record, we would only have been as good as yesterday's best."

O'Neill's commitment to safety paid off. During his last year at Alcoa, out of the entire 140,000 Alcoa employees worldwide, there were fewer than 15 incidents. Statistically, speaking, Alcoa had become a workplace where, on average, it would take 700 years before any individual would be subject to a lost workday because of an accident.

When he first came to the Pittsburgh Regional Health Initiative (PRHI), he was surprised to find that the lost workday rate in healthcare was 22 times worse than at Alcoa worldwide, even in plants "in countries where people claim they don't really value human life very much."

At PRHI, O'Neill asked a pharmacist to keep track for one day of all prescriptions received from doctors that required follow-up before they could be filled with confidence. Out of 150 prescriptions that day, the pharmacist had to make follow-up inquiries on 148. At that time, before the PRHI workers had learned systems thinking, pharmacists considered follow-up calls as a normal part of their job, and not as 148 errors and hours of wasted time. The pharmacists, once trained in process improvement, designed a standardized format and prescription form that reduced the need for follow-up calls by 50 percent.

When O'Neill came to PRHI, he brought the idea of the theoretical limit with him and began advocating it to the hospitals.

Without using that specific expression, Sister Mary Jean Ryan had also captured the same idea of defect-free health care in a system of hospitals, which she directed. SSM actually called their goal "Exceptional Healthcare" and aimed for the 99th percentile of perfection.

SETTING THEIR SIGHTS HIGH

In many organizations, leadership has given the idea of continual improvement an "easy" meaning—being content with a five- or ten-percent improvement in processes each year. At both PRHI and SSM Health Care, the leadership took a radical view of continual improvement. Instead of going for five percent, they asked, why not go for 100 percent? In other words, instead of being satisfied with reducing mistakes or waste by small percentage points each year, both health-care systems aimed at reducing errors or infection rates to zero as quickly as possible.

This theoretical limit approach gave great momentum for improvement in both healthcare systems, because it brought their long-term goal into focus.

> As regional vice president in the system I would review a lot of quality reports that came across my desk from 5 or 6 hospitals. The result was that I would see a report that would say we are at 95 percent compliance with a certain standard, no action necessary. And I would see that same comment month after month after month; everyone believed that 95 percent compliance was good enough and we would be very happy with that.
>
> I was dissatisfied with that personally and struggled for a way to get people to further commit.
>
> *William P. Thompson, Senior Vice President,*
> *Strategic Development, SSM Health Care*

If you walk around with Sister Mary Jean on a nursing division and they're looking at, say, improving patient satisfaction on this particular unit and it's at 95 percent, we have seen her actually challenge the people to go to 100 percent. People look at her like, "We can't get 100 percent." And she may agree that 100 percent is a stretch, but her mindset in terms of vision and foresight is, "Why not try for 100 percent or zero hospital-based infection rate?" I think that, at first, that kind of questioning and challenging caused everybody to open their eyes and wonder if this is really possible. Now you see people really focused on much greater stretch goals than we've ever had in the past.

William Schoenhard, Executive VP & COO,
SSM Health Care

Why not achieve the ideal? Why not have everybody in the Pittsburgh region receive 100 percent effective care as we know it? We need to identify what's keeping us from getting to the goal.

Tania Lyon, Ph.D., Chronic Care Coordinator,
PRHI

One of the models of thought that's been very, very helpful for us is to clearly define what the ideal is in any situation. For example, there will not be any medication errors; there will not be any nosocomial infections. Every patient that has diabetes or depression will have 100 percent effective treatment necessary for his or her disease state.

There are things that hold us back from those ideals. But by actually going for the ideal and then coming up to the barriers that keep us from those ideals, we can clearly define the counter measures necessary to get us closer and closer to the ideal. Perfection is not going to come easily, but perfection is something that can come, or at least can be approached incrementally by clearly defining the things that are keeping you from it.

The idea is to have a true understanding of where perfection exists, where the ideal is, and then you can move toward it. That's in chronic disease or any of our other clinical initiatives or safety initiatives.

Dennis Schilling, Clinical Coordinator,
PRHI

Our objective is perfect patient care. One of our goals is to actually pursue the goal of zero nosocomial infections. In other words, no one comes into this hospital as a patient and leaves with a pathogen or an infection that may damage their health. We do that by redesigning the work so it's both possible and easy for the healthcare workers here to follow the practices that prevent the spread of pathogens that make people sick.

Peter Perreiah, Director,
PRHI

I think you have to be a believer that you can have zero errors, be it readmissions, nosocomial infections, whatever the case may be. If you strive for it, I believe it can happen.

Connie Cibrone, President & CEO,
Allegheny General Hospital, PRHI

The term or the goal of zero infections is an ambitious goal, but it's very important to push the threshold, because how many infections are truly acceptable? If you truly believe in patient safety and perfecting patient care, not even one infection would be acceptable. So, when you're looking to redesign your system, you don't want to design your system to be 98 percent good, you want it to be 100 percent effective. Embracing that goal of zero infections, I believe, pushes everyone, challenges everyone to continue to work harder and harder to make sure that not one hospital-acquired infection happens.

Ellesha Miller, RN, Team Leader, PRHI,
VA Hospital Learning Alliance

I'd look to the federal government to do the things that are appropriate to it, but the really hard work—the getting it right at the point of care, patient by patient—that's a regional challenge that every region should step up to and meet.

Karen Wolk Feinstein, Chair & Founder, PRHI,
President, Jewish Healthcare Foundation

One of our goals at PRHI is to achieve zero defects. It's part of the Toyota Production System model that we're trying to apply to health care. That model can be perhaps more easily applied in a hospital setting where you can set goals like zero medication errors or zero nosocomial infections.

Tania Lyon, Ph.D., Chronic Care Coordinator,
PRHI

If you look at the products that come from Toyota, they pride themselves on quality and zero errors. And it's the same concept here. It's taking these tools and techniques and applying them to health care, where the idea is to have zero and the best outcomes. So, it's not like these principles are applicable only to a car or to somebody making a car, they are applicable to hospitals. I didn't think that way to begin with and actually went along with it because everybody seemed to be doing it. I didn't' really go in with an open mind.

Connie Cibrone, President & CEO,
Allegheny General Hospital, PRHI

Well, to take the principles we're trying to use to achieve the theoretical limit, they begin not with the Toyota Production System itself but with the idea of the ideal. This means understanding questions like, What do people need and are we meeting that need? And are we solving each specific problem to root cause as quickly as possible? We are proud to derive learning and a systems approach from the principles perfected by Toyota as a place that understands how to constantly improve how they meet customer need across a very complex task and organization by focusing on core principles and empowering everybody in the organization to act on them through a distinct design.

Kenneth Segel, former Executive Director,
PRHI

One of the core principles that empower everyone in the organization is to understand how to find the root cause of problems and why that is important. That's the next chapter.

Some Things to Remember From This Chapter

✔ The theoretical limit gives great momentum for improvement.

✔ The theoretical limit brings the long-term goal into focus.

✔ The theoretical limit is possible only in theory—100 percent perfection.

✔ Because of continual change and possibilities for improvement, the vision must be ever-flexible in using new information, skills and time.

✔ This allows the hospital to provide the best use of all resources and knowledge for the customer/patient at that moment.

✔ Perfect patient care if or when it can be achieved, will only last until new knowledge, new skills or new goals makes today or yesterday's perfection obsolete.

✔ Reaching zero errors is an important and necessary step toward the theoretical limit of "safest organization to work for" or "perfect patient care," but zero errors and the theoretical limit are not the same thing. The theoretical limit is an idea, e.g., "exceptional healthcare," that may change and develop with increasing knowledge and continual improvement.

CHAPTER 14

FINDING ROOT CAUSES
OF PROBLEMS

We would, as I mentioned earlier, inadvertently add additional complexity to the process. We would publish a new policy and procedure that had nothing to do with the root cause of the problem, and would only add to the complexity and confusion. The more you do that, the more you set up the potential for failure in providing the care directly to the patient. That may sound kind of ethereal, but it really does happen where nobody knows what happens. It becomes so complex that nobody has a clue of what all goes in to serving the patient. In many cases those well-intended additional policies and procedures were not enhancements but additions to the current process of care that only added more confusion and a likely set-up for medical accidents.

William Schoenhard, Executive VP & COO,
SSM Health Care

One of the biggest weaknesses of traditional linear thinking is the belief that every effect has an immediate cause, that is, that cause and effect are directly linked. In any organizations, when a problem is discovered, people ask, "Why is this happening?" and they look for a solution. They argue logically that every effect has a direct cause. They tend to focus on finding an immediate cause. In many cases, they identify the symptoms of the problem and try to remedy the symptoms, thinking thereby that they have solved the problem. (Much of medicine today follows this same path: focusing, not on getting to the root of a person's health problem, but on getting rid of its symptoms, usually the pain caused by the problem. This analogy, of course, doesn't apply when pain control is the only appropriate goal such as the last stages of terminal cancer.)

In contrast, in systems thinking, people are taught to dig more deeply to find the root cause of a problem. Systems thinkers have learned that cause and effect can be widely separated in time and space. For example, a child may be failing in school for causes that happened months or years ago, far from the classroom.

Toyota taught these healthcare professionals *not* to stop asking "Why?" after one "Why?" because most problems are deeper than they appear to be. Rather, to get to the root of many problems, Toyota's Production System said that one must ask "Why" four or five times, searching each time at a deeper level of the problem. Only when correcting the root cause of a problem will it be eliminated from the system.

This process of digging into root causes has been called the "Five Whys." The idea, when trying to solve a problem or find out why a mistake is happening, is to ask "Why?" once to find an immediate cause, then to ask "Why?" a second time to find the source of the immediate cause. When that source is found, ask "Why?" a third, a fourth, and even a fifth time, if necessary, to get to the root cause of the problem—its true source. Once the root cause is identified, whatever is causing the difficulty can be redesigned to prevent the problem from ever happening again.

In this chapter, personnel at PRHI and SSM Health Care tell how they learned to apply the "Five Whys" technique to find and resolve root causes of vexing problems such as broken medical carts, medical errors and confusingly dangerous written prescription abbreviations. For example, the time patients spent at the hospital registration desk—a bottleneck problem for most hospitals—was taking up to an hour. The staff used the Five Whys technique *many times over* in order to totally redesign the entire registration process and significantly reduce the time needed to complete it.

Case Study: Reducing Registration Time at PRHI

Hospital registration was taking about 12 minutes. One of the situations was that if three or four or five people would show up at the same time, which happened during certain times of the day, there was a huge backlog. People would wait over an hour, at times, to get registered. And sometimes they'd get frustrated.

So we studied this process. We applied the principles and we looked at value-added and non-value-added work and internal and external work as part of that process. I don't want to go on and on, but there were probably 20-to-30 changes that we made. Changes as small as putting little labels on people, and bins so people knew exactly where patients were, to larger changes in the way work was done and where it was done. But essentially, in the end, registration was taking only three minutes—and that's what it is today—instead of 12 minutes. It's quite amazing to see how quickly staff can work through a backlog of four or five patients showing up at the same time.

What's more important is that it can't go back to 12 minutes because the work design has been changed. That's one of the features about process improvement that I think is very interesting. It's not about checking up on people, it's not about telling people to be more careful or try to do a better job or make sure you remember this. Those things don't work. That's temporary stuff. But when you're actually changing the design of work, you're creating a place where people can come and do their best work and meet the needs of the patient, because that's the design.

David Sharbaugh, Director of Quality Improvement,
Shadyside Hospital, PRHI

It is a tremendous insight to realize that checking up on people or reminding them to do this or that is not an efficient way to improve a process or an employee's work. Only redesigning the process can build in improvement. This realization is a vitally important part of the mindset shift to systems thinking. Redesigning the process so that errors can't happen or steps can't be forgotten frees the staff to do their best work and meet the needs of the patients. Furthermore, the redesigned process keeps the staff from falling back into old ways or inadvertently making the registration process less efficient.

Everything we do, any change we make, anything we look at, immediately we're asking: How do we know if this is going to work? What can we do differently? If this isn't working, how should we change it? If it's doing well, can we do even better

168

the next time? And, if we do really well, can we share it with others or get some input from others? All this is just a part of what we do.

Diane Herbst, RN, Clinical Educator,
Critical Care Department, DePaul Health Center

Like human freedom, continual improvement demands "eternal vigilance."

The Five Whys technique, as well as other continual improvement tools, cannot be used sitting around a conference table, but must be practiced under workplace conditions where the problem is actually occurring. In order to achieve the theoretical limits of improvement in all areas, as many employees as possible need to be trained in this technique.

BEFORE THEY LEARNED SYSTEMS THINKING

In the past senior executives focused on outcomes rather than causes. Historically, we were focused on outcome measures only. There's not a lot you're going to do standing on the scale about what you weigh today. (Studying the process) may get around to caloric intake, exercise, fat content and the rest.

Now, we try to understand what those measures are around the major outcomes we're interested in and have those reflected in our departmental goals. Leaders are more and more focusing on those in-process measures, how well are we doing on our caloric intake and exercise routine as opposed to how much do we weigh today.

William Schoenhard, Executive VP & COO,
SSM Health Care

The teachings I have had actually helped me learn to look at the current condition and observe what's happening today. It helped me look at why things are happening. You may not understand a problem on the surface, but once you start asking a series of questions to probe the "why" of things, you may come to a different cause of the problem.

Ellesha Miller, RN, Team Leader, PRHI,
VA Hospital Learning Alliance

169

AN EXAMPLE OF FIVE WHYS: MEDICATION CARTS

The idea behind the Five Whys is to actually approach a problem that appears on the surface and ask why it occurred and to drill to the next level. A good example of this actually occurred on our medication carts. We had some very successful mistake-proofing done on these medication carts to eliminate breakdowns. We found that the batteries on these computers that were supporting our bar-code medication systems were often going dead. At first we suspected operator misuse, so we did some color-coding and labeling of buttons, some instructions in the local work area to make its use very easy and obvious.

One day we actually had a breakdown in the system. It didn't take long to solve the problem. The nurses worked right through the Five Whys, asking why did this go wrong. They found out in fact they had done everything right. They traced the problem back to the battery charger, which they found did not actually have any power. And when they asked why doesn't the battery charger have power, they found out that the electrical outlet was dead.

It turns out the outlet was located right next to a sink, and the outlet had been splashed with water, which tripped the ground fault, which turned off the outlet. When we asked why is water splashing on the outlet, we found the water pressure was too high in the sink. So, we called in the plumber. He adjusted the water pressure. We never had the outlet trip out again, and we no longer had that problem with the batteries.

By using this Five Whys technique over and over, we are able to uncover causes like the high water pressure that we never would have imagined to be the source in that system causing problems. And we were able to take care of that problem in a very efficient way. It doesn't take a lot of time or a lot of experts, for that matter, to do that kind of problem solving.

Peter Perreiah, Director,
PRHI

I have learned to see things from a much broader perspective. I have learned that problems that I thought were going on the surface were happening at a much deeper level, or seeing ways to improve things that I didn't even believe were a problem before.

Ellesha Miller, RN, Team Leader, PRHI,
VA Hospital Learning Alliance

EXAMPLES OF MEDICATION ERRORS

Looking for root causes for medication errors, pharmacy staff discovered that abbreviations for drugs, handwritten on prescriptions were easily misread.

One of the other main focuses of our medication safety team was looking at dangerous abbreviations that doctors and other healthcare professionals use.

One of the most dangerous abbreviations is using the little *u* for designating units, because a sloppily written *u* can look like a *0*, a *4* or a *6*. Suddenly a four-unit "4u" dose of insulin becomes 44 or a 6 unit dose "6u" becomes 60 so we're looking at potentially ten-fold or greater doses, doses that can kill our patients. We're trying to take good care of our patients by using abbreviations that are appropriate. I tell everybody: start with the *u*; get rid of that one abbreviation from your medical vocabulary first.

Another was a medication that's fairly new. The physician who had prescribed it probably wasn't familiar with it either. And because it was something I don't normally dispense, I looked up the medication and found that he had dosed it incorrectly. In that case, a simple phone call fixed it. Sometimes, it's not that easy. Sometimes these things get past us. The days when the safety net is not there are when we notice all the holes in the Swiss cheese. The wrong prescription gets past one safety barrier after another, and it makes it all the way through to the patient. Those are the bad days when all the holes line up.

Chris Grass, Clinical Pharmacist,
SSM DePaul Health Center

THE NUN AND THE BUREAUCRAT

In the patient safety collaborative we've seen a 50 percent reduction in dangerous abbreviations.

An example would be a physician's order of medication for a patient using abbreviations that have been standardized over the years of health care. The healthcare industry is learning that some of those abbreviations can lead to misinterpretation and an error on a medical prescription. For example QD means "every day" (from the Latin *quotidie*). A physician might write an order that a patient is to receive X medication QD: every day. That abbreviation can be misinterpreted, and that could lead to a misdose being given to a patient.

The Q could look like an O or the D could look like an O. If the writing is not legible, then that could lead to an inaccurate dose being given to the patient or the medication being given at a frequency that is not correct.

Another example of a dangerous abbreviation is the decimal point. Say, we want the dose to be ten units of a medication. If the physician writes a decimal point and then adds a zero following it, it could be misinterpreted as 100 units. So, we're working with our facilities to eliminate those *trailing* zeros and promote the use of *leading* zeros. If a medication dose needs to be .2, we put a zero in front of the 2 *[0.2]*. Then it's very clear what the dose should be.

IDENTIFYING EASILY CONFUSED DRUGS

We're learning that a lot of drugs are packaged in similar looking packages. Or their names may sound similar. We call these "look alike" or "sound alike" medications, and we're working with the suppliers to change the packaging. For example, if we have two medications packaged in a syringe with a yellow label, we ask that they change the color of those labels, so we can't confuse the two medications.

Shelley Niemeyer, Quality Resource Center Consultant,
SSM Health Care

We have become much more proactive, rather than reactive. We're trying to fix problems before they occur. I think that has resulted in a dramatic improvement in the organization.

Kevin Johnson, MD, VP for Medical Affairs,
SSM DePaul Health Center

We have started a procedure called two-patient identifiers, so that when we give our medications we have a computerized med sheet in our hands. We take this med sheet with us to the patient's room, and the patient has an ID bracelet with both his name and his birth date. We ask them to tell us their name and their birth date. And then also we check to see if they have an allergy band on and verify on our med sheet that whatever allergies they may have are also printed there. So, today we're checking all this before we give medicines.

Patricia Abramczyk, RN, Staff Nurse, Orthopedics,
SSM DePaul Health Center

Our significant medication error rate for 2002 was 0.16 per thousand dosages administered. Our second quarter this year, it is 0.01 per thousand—sixteen time better. We dramatically improved things. A lot of that is attributed to our continuous quality improvement culture, the way we aggressively analyze problems and issues, and strive to implement change or action plans to get to the results we want.

Kevin Johnson, MD, VP for Medical Affairs,
SSM DePaul Health Center

SIMPLIFYING A CONFUSING PHARMACY ENVIRONMENT

A hospital pharmacy is a rather chaotic environment and for a pharmacist to enter orders it's very confusing at times. There are a lot of distractions in this process. We found, through our real time reporting, that this has led to some errors. So we created a distraction-free area. There a pharmacist can be focused on entering the orders without telephones ringing and without people interrupting him with questions.

We're experimenting with one unit doing the scan-to-email process. In the past we've had to fax our orders downstairs, and the faxes are often difficult to read, let alone when you're trying to interpret a physician's questionable handwriting. So, by doing the scan-to-email we get a better quality picture of the order that's actually written upstairs. It's displayed on the computer here in the pharmacy.

On the one unit where we've begun using this, since the middle of August, we have dramatically reduced the number of medication errors related to the earlier fax process.

Elaine Hatfield, MPM, Clinical Operations Officer
LifeCare Hospitals of Pittsburgh, PRHI

However continual improvement never ends.

If you ask me about the cost of medical errors in our hospital that do reach the patient, I don't have a figure for you, but it's significant... Even if an error doesn't harm the patient significantly, there is a major cost with increasing the length of stay, monitoring blood, other testing, and a variety of other medications that you use in an adverse event. The cost is very high.

JoAnn V. Narduzzi, MD, Ph.D., VP of Academic Affairs,
Pittsburgh Mercy Health System, PRHI

An obvious method for insuring that the correct prescription gets from the doctor to the pharmacy and to the right patient or keeping track of the proper doses for patients of various weights and ages would be to use computers. Some hospitals are buying computers for everything from identifying patients with wristbands to prescriptions and detailed patient records. They can also be used to monitor patients at the bedside.

Some large medical systems, from the Veteran's Administration Hospitals to HMOs, are beginning to install expensive and extensive computer programs, and errors are being reduced.

However, it is important to remember that computers are only tools and not only can't substitute for systems knowledge, but can give healthcare personnel a false sense of security.

The computer "is not a cookbook that tells you what to do," said Eugene Wiener, MD, medical director of Children's Hospital. "Instead it asks you to consider: Did you know this? Did you think about that?"

Many doctors are reluctant to use computers except for billing. A CDC report in 2005 indicated that while 73 percent of doctors' offices use computer technology for billing, just 17 percent use it to maintain records and only 8 percent to order prescriptions electronically, according to *The Pittsburgh Post-Gazette.*

Using computers as a management tool in a complex hospital environment requires extensive and deep training. Like other advances in technology that allow people to live longer and be sicker, the computer offers paradoxical advantages and disadvantages.

There are always more opportunities for safe-proofing the system so errors will not occur. Protocols and checklists at SSM and PRHI have been a significant factor in delivering better, safer care and freeing doctors and nurses to have more time with the patient. We examine those next.

SOME THINGS TO REMEMBER FROM THIS CHAPTER

✓ Cause and effect may be widely separated in time and space.

✓ The ultimate cause may not be what it first seems to be, e.g., the water pressure in a nearby sink is the cause of the malfunctioning medical cart.

✓ Ask "Why?" five times to find causes and make effective improvements and solve problems.

✓ Redesigning processes safeguards improvements and frees staff to meet the needs of patients.

✓ Computers can be helpful, but operators need systems knowledge, particularly in a complex hospital.

CHAPTER FOOTNOTES

[1] PRHI Executive Summary Report, February 2004, page 2, Pittsburgh, PA.

CHAPTER 15

USING PROTOCOLS
AND CHECKLISTS

If we fixed the system itself, I don't think the employee would make the error. I truly don't. You know, if we had fail-safe procedures, just like they do in the aerospace industry where they have to have these things in place, or else planes would be crashing every day.

Christine Quinn, Director of Professional Service,
LifeCare Hospitals of Pittsburgh, PRHI

TRANSLATING THE VISION INTO ACTION

Hospital leadership must take the first steps to transform the organization, as we said earlier. They must commit to improvement and identify a unifying purpose to which all employees can readily commit such as "perfect patient care" or continual improvement.

However, once the vision is established, it needs to be translated into the hospital's daily work with patients. This translation of idea into action is the work best done by employees in each unit. Their challenge is to find ways to realize the vision in the course of activity throughout the hospital. It's no small matter—or more precisely, it involves thousands of small matters.

Once employees are aligned in pursuit of the vision the hard work begins. Problems must be identified. Solutions must be tested. Conflicts must be resolved. Processes must be improved. Missing procedures must be introduced. These changes are not the work of a moment, but require painstaking observation, precise data gathering, exploratory meetings, mapping of flow charts, and suggested re-designs, which must be tested, then tweaked, adjusted and refined, before they can be standardized.

In the previous chapter we saw how the people at PRHI and SSM Health Care used various Toyota and systems thinking methods to get to the roots of problems and re-design work so that these problems would not occur again.

In this chapter we get to see the creative side of the systems-thinking mind at work in originating protocols and checklists for use in the emergency department, cardiac units, surgical theaters, isolation rooms, and for supply inventories throughout the hospital.

Within any big organization like a hospital with its many complex procedures, the staff cannot be expected to remember to do everything every time. Allowing for inevitable human error, these two healthcare systems realized they had to create fail-safe processes where errors would be unlikely to occur. They researched each process and created checklists to ensure that no steps or details are omitted. Often these procedures are done with a "pilot-copilot" format, where the copilot follows the pilot's actions using a checklist.

SSM Health Care, which has been addressing such problems for many more years than PRHI, found that most patients come to hospital emergency rooms with one of a small range of common diseases— about 20 to 30 of them. Protocols, or lists of procedures to treat each of these diseases, have been developed and approved by the physicians, so the staff is authorized to follow them. It is a form of "safe proofing" the treatment of patients. And it also saves valuable time for medical personnel and patients.

Standard procedures based on extensive data about best practices and outcomes can prevent errors before they occur. This is called evidence-based medicine. It is different and more effective than old practices where individual doctors relied on their medical school learning and their personal experience with the individuals they treated.

> I think that the old culture, so to speak, was where physicians were practicing medicine in some isolation…they would use their anecdotal experience to treat the next patient because that was the best evidence they had to go on. So, when they were successful using a treatment for one patient they would use it for another. Gradually, it has become clear that for certain conditions there are what we call evidence-based interventions, or therapies that can be adopted for most patients.

It's been a gradual change and it's a remarkable change in health care now—the shift from physicians practicing individually and not having frequent dialogues with other colleagues about the processes of care, to making some standardization of care, protocols and pathways that we use in the care of patients.

The more we can make the more routine types of patient care standardized, the more chance physicians and other caregivers have to spend the time that they need on other, particularly difficult situations, where both time and resources are needed and aren't easily amenable to any kind of standardization.

Andrew Kosseff, MD, Director, Clinical Systems Improvement
SSM Health Care

We're trying to make sure that we treat all of our patients who suffer from these various conditions according to evidence-based medicine, and have it standardized and systematized across the organization.

For example, we're making sure that we have surgical site marking on all surgeries where the patient and the physician agree that this is the right side to do surgery on. It sounds relatively simple, but there have been errors across the country because of mistakes around that issue. We're taking "time outs" before surgery. We're doing projects to make sure we have accurate medication lists. We're improving some of the technology around medication distribution. It's a series of things. But we're working on them one by one across our hospitals. And we're showing a lot of improvement.

Paul Convery, MD, Chief Medical Officer
SSM Health Care/St. Louis

THE AIRLINE EXAMPLE

In the airline industry they recognize human beings can make mistakes and they have really intensive checklists. They build in a human factor and a mechanical factor that makes it much, much more difficult to make an error.

We want to try to provide healthcare workers with an environment conducive to good quality care where they do not have to second-guess themselves and do not have the potential for making errors.

This is what we have to continue to do in health care. One of the principles I've learned in perfecting patient care is to make sure people can't do the wrong thing.

How do you make that happen, how do you make sure people do the right thing? There's a lot of redundancy built in, steps that work.

Deborah Thompson, RN, Quality Trainer,
PRHI

ERRORS OF OVERSIGHT

Hospital care is complex and the errors we make are frequently errors of oversight. We forget to do things because of a lack of structure. Physicians like to be independent thinkers. Every one of them was at the top of their class when they got out of high school and college. And they really feel that they have all the answers. They're very, very bright and talented people but they get distracted. I think bringing structure to care in the hospital will help amazingly.

We have over 30 order sets for the common diseases that bring structure to each treatment plan, to try and prevent folks, really very good and talented people, from making simple errors of oversight. Forgetting that a patient is allergic to something or forgetting to prescribe treatment for deep venous thrombosis prophylaxis, these blood clots that form in people's legs and migrate to the lungs and kill them in the hospital. Virtually every patient is at risk for that, but we don't in every instance remember to prescribe for it.

So we have instituted a program here where the case managers go through the charts of patients who aren't on prophylaxis and put a reminder sticker in the chart. You really want that reminder up front, and structured order sets for doctors. Computerized physician order entry with little reminders built into them will, I think, go a long way to improving inpatient care.

It's dotting the i's and crossing the t's that saves a great number of lives in the hospital. Most people have common diseases for which we have common and very effective treatments.

Filippo Ferrigni, MD, VP, Critical Care Director
SSM St. Joseph's Health Center

Once the diagnosis has been determined, we have developed the best protocols for treatment to achieve the maximum outcome. And also we know more and more, as we learn patient safety practices, how care can be delivered in a safer environment.

William Schoenhard, Executive VP & COO,
SSM Health Care

We've had a collaborative around congestive heart failure for sharing improvements of therapy. That's an ongoing collaborative for improvements in treatment of ischemic heart disease.

They are focused on implementing evidence-based improvements in care. Some of it is recent. Unfortunately, some of it is evidence that's ten, 15 years old, but it's still not widespread in medical practice.

For example, there's been evidence for a number of years that treating all patients with acute myocardial infarctions with aspirin and beta blocker will decrease mortality and morbidity. When you test physicians on that knowledge, they all test very highly. They've read a number of articles that relate to that. When you look at their patients and their charts, you don't find that kind of compliance. So it's not a knowledge gap.

Paul Convery, MD, Chief Medical Officer
SSM Health Care/St. Louis

Over the last two years we have dramatically improved our performance. An example of that would be giving aspirin in the emergency room for an acute myocardial infarction. When we first started measuring our performance, we were probably 40 to 50 percent compliant. And now we're 95 to 98 percent compliant.

Kevin Johnson, MD, VP for Medical Affairs,
SSM DePaul Health Center

We have to put processes in place for the nurses, even under times of stress, so that errors don't occur.

JoAnn V. Narduzzi, MD, Ph.D., VP of Academic Affairs,
Pittsburgh Mercy Health System, PRHI

Making sure people can't do the wrong thing.

Deborah Thompson, RN, Quality Trainer,
PRHI

The complexities of taking care of the patients can be so overwhelming. There are so many things going on at the same time. There's so many different demands that it's really beyond the capability of even very bright, well-intentioned people to remember every single detail. And so you have to build it into the systems that remind them of the detail or alerts them to the possibility of ordering the aspirin and beta blocker.

Paul Convery, MD, Chief Medical Officer
SSM Health Care/St. Louis

PROTOCOLS AND PROCEDURES IN THE SUPPLY STATIONS

Some of the most effective improvements in hospitals are not necessarily dramatic ones, as in marking the proper limb for surgery or prescribing the correct medication. Rather, they include things like streamlining housekeeping methods and inventory-keeping, so that sterile gowns and gloves are always at hand when needed, and other supplies are always in stock, so a nurse doesn't have to leave a patient to search for a fresh bandage. Here, the Toyota inventory control system helped hospitals create new ways of stocking supplies, which led to a significant drop in hospital-acquired infections and medical errors, many of which could prove fatal to patients.

Patients are not cars. We are dealing with patients, each of whom is a unique case. Standard practices that have a lot of variation in them. So initially, I wasn't sure how it would end up.

It's very hard to standardize processes with people. But after learning that the Toyota Production System was all about understanding your current condition, we found lots of things we can improve and standardize.

I must say, after two years, I am impressed with the job that we have been able to do. And I believe that we can go a lot further in improving the patient care system using these techniques.

For example, before, it was everyone's responsibility to make sure that gowns and gloves needed for isolation precautions were available. We were able to standardize the system and make it one person's responsibility to routinely check the shelves every day to always make sure that supplies are available.

Under the old system, if you used the last gown you were supposed to call and get a new gown. But that approach may generate waste or make patients wait, as you waited for your equipment to come to you. But through the new system, we are actually able to meet patients' needs without any interruptions or waste.

Ellesha Miller, RN, Team Leader, PRHI,
VA Hospital Learning Alliance

The VA also reorganized its isolation anteroom where doctors and nurses get themselves ready to step into an isolation room.

The purpose of this room is for people to come in and put on the proper protective equipment before taking care of a patient who might be in isolation or carrying a specific organism. These rooms were designed with cupboards that hold isolation supplies. So we standardized or stabilized our system. We were able to spell out each item that needed to be in this cupboard. Things are color-coded and we have a designated supplier. So now the nursing assistant supplies everything in this cupboard that is labeled with blue.

Through study of the situation and calculations, we're now certain there are enough supplies here to last for a 24-hour period. Every day at 7 am, our nursing assistant comes in and checks supplies. It's very interesting, the design of the system, because it tells you exactly on the back of the cupboard how many of what items are supposed to be there. So the assistants know exactly what equipment they are supposed to replace every day. There's no question and no ambiguity in the system. And there is no waste because you are not counting unneeded supplies.

We took this idea from manufacturing to improve patient care and we have what we call safety stock. In the event our system becomes unstable for a day or a couple of hours, patient care will still go on. You still have your needed equipment.

Ellesha Miller, RN, Team Leader, PRHI,
VA Hospital Learning Alliance

Even small changes, like putting up coat hooks in the isolation anteroom, made big differences in efficiency and effectiveness.

Through talking to doctors and nurses we recognized that... they didn't want to wear their hospital lab coat over a gown into a patient's room. Coats over gowns really didn't fit well. A small thing like putting up hooks to hold the residents' lab coats has made a great improvement. That way the residents can be compliant with the precautions, and not have to take their own excess equipment into the patient's room. They can lay their stethoscopes in the room and other items that they don't want to take into the resistant organism rooms. The true beauty of the Toyota Production System is its focus on: How do you make it easier for people do to the work the right way and not really have to leave the point of patient care?

The true benefits are for our patients who don't have to wait because of a delay in here. Under the old system, if you used the last gown and needed to order a gown, you may have had to wait a few minutes for those supplies to come before you could actually go in and provide patient care. Patients no longer have to *wait* for care. It's actually a lot easier to find things, too. You don't have to look through different cupboards to find what you need. It's spelled out. The nursing staff knows what they need and they know where it's supposed to be. So, there's a reliability that it's always there.

One of the other things is the huge push of our project to enable people to embrace infection-control precautions. It's very important to always have the supplies that you need so that you always do the right thing for a patient, and not transmit hospital-acquired infections.

Ellesha Miller, RN, Team Leader, PRHI,
VA Hospital Learning Alliance

Pursuing continual improvement in treatment and supplies is a general goal SSM has learned over the years in its many facilities. However, implementation is local and success is creating a self-organizing system.

Now there are a lot of issues around standardization, centralization, variation and diversification and all that sort of thing. And we're constantly testing the limits and the balance between what we're doing as a larger system and what individual hospitals are doing, but for the most part I think we've reached a very comfortable balance. Responsible for the large system, we in leadership have to set the general direction and the parameters, but health care is truly delivered on a local basis so we allow the system to become self-organizing to meet the needs of each local community.

William P. Thompson, Senior Vice President,
Strategic Development, SSM Health Care

There will be more about self-organization and checklists in the next chapter where in one unit frontline workers reduced the number of frequently fatal infections to zero.

SOME THINGS TO REMEMBER FROM THIS CHAPTER

✓ Healthcare delivery has become so complex that staff cannot be expected to remember every detail every time.

✓ It is possible to set up a fail-safe way to help people avoid mistakes.

✓ Protocols and checklists are two effective tools for doing this.

✓ A pilot/copilot format for guiding personnel through complex procedures is also powerful.

✓ These methods not only insure safe treatment, they save time and eliminate ambiguity, a frequent and hidden cause of serious hospital error.

✓ Careful observation of how treatment is given, reliable distribution of supplies needed for successful treatment, and continual improvement of safe methods are the underlying supports of perfect patient care.

CHAPTER 16

EMPOWERING FRONTLINE WORKERS

We very much believe in decision making at the low-est point possible in an organization. It's a concept of subsidiarity where those that are most impacted and those that are involved helped to make the decisions in terms of how things are structured.

Paula Friedman, Vice President, Systems Improvement, SSM Health Care

Traditionally, quality control professionals were called in to study problems of patient infection or patient mortality. The expert team would collect data over an extended period, study and summarize their research, then make suggestions for improvement. This procedure sometimes took as long as six months to a year. At SSM and PRHI, they have changed much of that practice. Today, they do what is called *real-time problem solving*.

Real-time problem solving was developed at Toyota where workers who spot a problem on the assembly line can pull an emergency cord and stop the entire line to make even a minor adjustment. This was revolutionary when Toyota began to allow it in the mid 20th Century. Workers in traditional auto plants then did what they were told and didn't volunteer suggestions for improvement, much less stop the sacred assembly line.

As soon as a problem occurs at PRHI hospitals, the front-line workers analyze what went wrong and propose a solution, which is tested as soon as possible. If this solution resolves the problem so that it cannot occur again, the change is formally implemented throughout a department and, ultimately, the entire hospital. If the problem still occurs, another change in the process is tested until a true solution is found. Sometimes, problems are solved in one day.

SSM has developed its own method over the years and calls it

"Shared Accountability." Whatever it is called, it saves lives, reduces suffering and waste and allows the front-line medical personnel to take satisfaction and joy as they contribute to improving patient care.

Front-line people can solve problems because they have become systems thinkers. They can recognize whether or not a suggested change would truly be an improvement of the system.

In this chapter you will read how the leadership at both PRHI and SSM Health Care discovered the creative power and potential of front-line hospital staff to solve problems, even across departments. One story is about creating a new "supporting nurse" function on patient units—a person whose job it is to see that all 40 or more items required in every patient's room are always ready and available for use. Another account tells of solving the complaints of hungry patients waiting hours for a meal after their physician has approved a change of diet. Finally, we let people at PRHI tell the amazing story of how front-line nurses helped not only to significantly decrease the number of central line infections occurring among patients but also to reduce to zero in 90 days fatalities due to those infections.

By the way, veteran Toyota workers report that over the years they spot more and more problems, because they have learned how to "see" better and better.

> It's all about looking. Observing. Does the patient get the medicine when they need it? Do they get the right medicine at the closest time? How do we insure supplies are there? How do we insure that we have time to do the right things for patients?
>
> How you learn is by going and looking and seeing, being focused on solving the problem—trying a solution, changing that solution. And, if it doesn't work, trying another solution.
>
> *Deborah Thompson, RN, Quality Trainer,*
> *PRHI*

> Before now, nurses would just go through the routine. If they did not get a medication on time from the pharmacy, they would be frustrated and they would continue to make their phone calls or follow whatever process it took to get that medication.

They would still be frustrated and upset and they would be angry. But most importantly, the patient wasn't getting what the patient needed.

Tina Danzuso, RN, Ward Director General Surgery,
Shadyside Hospital, PRHI

With our learning line we've tackled a lot of issues with the staff. One that made a huge difference in everyone's mind was this process of signing in and signing out narcotics. Somewhere along the line, the pharmacy guides and nursing guides all got together and said, "Even though someone counted them downstairs, and someone else double counted them, you have to come upstairs and you have to count them in front of another nurse. You then have to put them in a machine that counts them every time you pull one out."

On average, this re-counting consumes about 17 minutes per unit. Knowing this, the minute a nurse would see the pharmacy person coming to re-count drugs that had been counted ten times before, she would run and hide or make excuses. "Oh I'm busy. I don't have time for you right now."

All this counting and hunting has been a big issue, so I picked up the phone and called the director of pharmacy. I could see all this with my own eyes through the staff. I said, "If you're counting meds this many times in the pharmacy, why does the nurse have to count them again when we put them in a machine that also electronically counts. I can't get a drug out unless I put my number in. So, why do we count again, and why are we wasting this much time, and why are we frustrating your employee who is chasing a nurse who doesn't want to take time away from a patient? Why are we doing this?"

The answer came back, "Well, we've always been worried if we were ever going to lose a narcotic."

And I asked, "Well, have we ever lost one? Have we ever had narcotics stolen from this process?"

The reply, "No, not that I can remember in my 25 years."

"Well then why are we doing it?"

"Well, just 'cause we have."

"So, can we stop it?"

"Yes, okay."

So we stopped it the next day. You know, that's a classic example of an old system that had just layered technology on without taking away the past.

Tami Merryman, RN, Vice President, Patient Care Service,
Shadyside Hospital, PRHI

Another lesson here was how much time could be saved and improvement made with an open mind and a single telephone call.

EMPOWERING FRONT-LINE WORKERS

What we're trying to do at SSM is to say to people, "We know that there are a lot of things that don't work very well, but we also know that there are people who are engaged in these activities who know how to fix these things better than we do." But it isn't just a department. Often it is a process that cuts across all departments. So, we tell them, "Put some people together, work on this and make it better, because when you make it better for the patient, you will also make it better for yourself."

What we are trying to say to people is, "Look, we know that you're bright, you're committed, you're dedicated to this, and you really want to make things better for the people that we serve. You know how to do what it takes to get this thing done. We'll train you to work through this whole process and then you'll have the authority to make these changes."

Sister Mary Jean Ryan, FSM, RN, President & CEO,
SSM Health Care

What we're trying to do is unleash the creativity and innovation of all people involved in our ministry who know best how to improve the care where they deliver the care. It may be right

189

at the bedside if they're a direct patient care deliverer. It may be in the support position in the laundry or in central supply.

The people who work with these processes every day know best how they can be improved, to ultimately serve the patient and the family of the patient. That, in a nutshell, is what we're about. We don't expect everybody to understand all the science of quality improvement. But we would expect everyone to understand our mission and the way they directly contribute to improving care consistent with our mission each day.

William Schoenhard, Executive VP & COO,
SSM Health Care

The idea, then, is to take the people who have the most insight about the way work is designed and focus on very small problems and redesign the work so that these problems do not creep in and become very large problems.

Peter Perreiah, Director,
PRHI

SHARED ACCOUNTABILITY

Our shared accountability model. That's where we involve the staff in decision-making on an everyday basis and ask them to participate in that decision-making.

Maggie Fowler, Vice President of Patient Services
SSM St. Joseph's Health Center

Shared accountability is really a philosophy and a way that the nurses do their work. They can be other professionals as well, pharmacists, lab techs, anybody who touches the patient. But the whole thought is that, since they are the people who are providing the care, why shouldn't they have more say in their schedule and in the way the care is rendered? Shared accountability is a structure that is set up within hospitals, run by council members, and those council members are the staff nurses. The shift in thinking doesn't happen overnight. It takes a long time to change that whole way of providing care to the patients.

> _Eunice Halverson, Corporate Vice President_
> _Quality Resource Center, SSM Health Care_

We had a facility in Madison, Wisconsin, St. Mary's Hospital Medical Center, that introduced this concept of shared accountability. It was a recognition that within the profession of nursing, since nurses were responsible for the delivery of care to patients, therefore, they should be the ones who have the authority to make changes in the care delivery process. This is going back to some of our original values of subsidiarity, of pushing decisions down to the most appropriate level.

One of the things they did there was to share not only clinical information but also financial and strategic and other information, so that the nurses had all the information needed to make appropriate decisions.

As a result, at St. Mary's we had some of the highest, most satisfied nursing professionals, the lowest turnover rates, and the lowest vacancy rate. But we also were discovering we had some of the highest and best clinical outcomes as well as some of the lowest costs of any provider in the state of Wisconsin. We decided as a system that we would take that demonstrated best practice and make it a requirement across our entire system.

> _William P. Thompson, Senior Vice President,_
> _Strategic Development, SSM Health Care_

This example, like the earlier one of the blood sugar lowering in the ICU, demonstrates the value of SSM's system where such innovations can be spread easily because of CQI culture.

THE SUPPORT NURSING ASSISTANT

We worked on creating a person called a support nursing assistant whose main function is to support the in-room patient caregivers by making sure their supplies are there, by using a supply ticket system, by making sure that the supply room is

191

up to date and has the supplies that they need to care for the 40 variations of care needs in these patient rooms. They make sure the hallways look clean and welcoming for visitors and patients, so they're not walking through a landmine of mess. The support aide relieves and creates some cushion for the clinical staff to stay in the rooms with the patients.

We did a lot of work doing these hour-by-hour observations, identifying facts about how much time is actually spent with the patient—how much in direct care and how much time in indirect care, which is outside of the room, hunting, fetching, and looking for things. Especially how much is literally just wasteful work. We started to get rid of the waste. Then we started to ask, "What actually are the steps in the indirect work in caring for patients and do they all make sense? Do we really need to do this?" Very often, the answer was no.

Susan Christie Martin, RN, Director, Nursing Support Services,
Shadyside Hospital, PRHI

FEEDING PATIENTS

What we didn't know is that between 6:00 and 7:00 in the morning 22 surgeons have made their rounds and left behind a huge bowl of medical orders, half of which were diet advances, such as, give this patient a soft tray. Maybe many of those patients haven't eaten in days. Perhaps cranberry juice or something from the fixings cupboard would be very refreshing for them to have because they would have to wait sometimes 2 or 3 hours to get their diet advance. By the subsidiarity initiative that we put on, using the diet hostess, we improved her skills to be able to review medical charts and look for diet advances that could be implemented immediately. This really elevated her as a participant in caring for this patient by actually seeing what the diet order for this patient is and going to the kitchen to fix it on demand, when the patient needs it. I can feel very proud of that.

Susan Christie Martin, RN, Director, Nursing Support Services,
Shadyside Hospital, PRHI

They discovered there was often at least a two-hour turn-around time between the doctor's visit to the patient, when the new order was written and processed, the tray was made in the kitchen, and it was delivered to the patient. By the time those two hours were up, the patients were very dissatisfied. The diet hostess explains:

> My responsibility is to make sure the patients are always satisfied with each meal and that they get their food on time, especially on time. In this little kitchen off the nurses' station, I make sure all the drawers are clean and the supplies are in place.
>
> Before, our patients used to wait half an hour to 45 minutes for a tray. They no longer have to wait that long now. Since I'm here, they wait only 5 to 10 minutes.
>
> Before, we had to wait for a phone call from downstairs, and then they'd get back to us through the computer. It used to be very, very tricky to get food out there.
>
> We have actually made my job easier because our patients are more satisfied. Prior to having these late trays supplied on the floor, we would get a lot of complaints. Because this delay has diminished, the patients are a lot happier. They get food immediately, when they're hungry—as soon as we get word of their order. Also, the hostesses are happier because they are meeting the patient's needs earlier as well.
>
> Until we learned to observe—how to "root cause" things—we really weren't getting to the bottom of the problems at all.
>
> *Lacy Peterson, Dietician,*
> *Shadyside Hospital, PRHI*

FEELING EMPOWERED TO MAKE CHANGES

Health professionals are deluged with data. So, to give them a bit of information about the number of people who got X infection in the last six months in their unit is not going to bring about behavior change. Telling them real stories of how various units have erased central line infections or giving them concrete examples of how they can get close to perfect performance in any one item is really more important than giving them more data. Not that you can separate the two. The data, the evidence foundation, is important.

Karen Wolk Feinstein, Chair & Founder, PRHI,
President, Jewish Healthcare Foundation

Prior to the partnership with PRHI, many of us felt that we didn't have the tools and we certainly didn't feel that we were empowered to do the work. Now, nurses are engaged and energized by the ability every day to make sure an error doesn't happen. And that's a tremendous liberating feeling for a nurse who otherwise comes to work every day trying to do the right thing but oftentimes finds herself inadvertently in circumstances where the system creates barriers to the proper care. So, that's what PRHI has done on a regional basis.

If you don't empower everyone who is involved in the process of delivering care and delivering care in the most effective way, then what you'll have is a malfunctioning system populated by people who are alienated from the very thing that they're trying to get done.

Richard Shannon, MD, Chairman, Department of Medicine,
Allegheny General Hospital, PRHI

CENTRAL LINE INFECTIONS

Dr. Shannon tells the compelling story of how frontline workers virtually eliminated a complex problem with central line infections which had caused much death, suffering and cost.

The challenge in our institution was that PRHI had asked each of the institutions in western Pennsylvania to commit to reducing hospital-acquired infections, by whatever amount they decided, over the course of the next year. Our institution thought it was boldly proclaiming that we would reduce central line infections by 50 percent in the next year.

The usual approach would be to call the quality management committee and the critical care committee together, to collect all the people in these committees that aren't operating at the bedside and say, "Okay, what are we going to do to reduce this?"

The approach we took was different. We said, "We're going to look at every one of these infections as they occur in real time and see if we can eliminate them in 90 days."

This was not the first attempt to reduce infections, but they found that the nature of the historical data researchers gave them, for example, in the form of bar graphs and other statistics, concealed rather than revealed useful information about fixing the problem. PRHI, through the Toyota Production System, showed them a different way to approach the problem. As Dr. Shannon explains,

> For 18 months, we had collected data that demonstrated a certain grade of infection in our ICUs. Historically, what happens with that data is it's shared in the form of bar graphs and lines that really don't convey the personal nature of what these infections are all about.
>
> Rather, these data conceal the fact and insulate us, particularly when they're reported after the fact and far from the reality of what is really patient safety and how important it is. It's about the people. Medical errors, unlike clinical outcomes, are really loaded with emotion.
>
> What PRHI has taught us is actually to come to the bedside, to engage the patient, to understand the processes of care that go into placing the central line, and really determine at root cause in real time why a line becomes infected. So, together with the nurses here in the ICU who have done this work, we have developed countermeasures to guarantee that lines are examined each day, that they're addressed in a standard fashion, and that when a line infection develops we actually have the opportunity to come right away and determine why the infection occurred.
>
> By doing that, two things happen. One is you get new learning. Discovering why this line became infected allows us to immediately change the process, so it won't happen again. Secondly,

you are forced to engage the patient who is the real centerpiece of this complication. When you do that, I think there's a real reinforcement about why we want to eliminate infections.

Dr. Shannon explains what a central line infection is and how the central lines work.

> Just briefly, central line infections occur as a consequence of placing lines in several large veins, usually in the neck. They are associated with an astonishing morbidity and mortality. It is a morbidity and mortality that would never be apparent from the sort of data reporting that you typically see. More importantly, these infections are preventable. The difference between this front-line approach and the quarterly cost-view approach is that we do real-time rates of infection.

> When an infection occurs, we actually try to understand in real time what happened. It's a critical factor that allows us to develop countermeasures based upon intense observation, not based upon guesses. So, looking at infections in real time, as opposed to reviewing them on a quarterly basis, allows you to create countermeasures and immediately address the underlying root cause, not three months from now but immediately.

> Here is an example. Frequently, patients have central lines placed in their femoral vein, which we learned by observation were associated with a higher risk of infections We simply asked physicians from then on to avoid using the femoral vein where possible, and to put the central line in a subclavian vein, which our experience, as well as the national experience, would suggest has a lower rate of infection. So, now we have many more lines in place in the subclavian position. With that counter-measure alone, we dramatically reduced the rate of infection.

> While the problem seems daunting at first, when you look at it in terms of bar graphs and data, if you take each infection one at a time and solve it to root cause, you can actually overcome these very significant infections—and in this case in 90 days.

THE NURSES DID IT

A couple of other points to mention. Nurses do this work; it's not done by physicians. We work together to try and create the working construct for doing this. These nurses taught us how to change a dressing. They taught us what the best practice is for doing that. They taught us how to examine a line to determine when it might need to be removed. We asked the nurses to prompt the doctors when they thought a line should come out. We asked the nurses to ask the doctors each day if they really needed this line any longer.

Our nursing IV team has developed a peripheral IV access that can sometimes replace these central lines and reduce the infection rate. So, the other interesting thing about this work is that it's really done by nurses. It's not done by physicians. As we physicians engage nurses doing the work of care, we learn all kinds of new things, as opposed to the historical practice of some committee telling them how to do their work. That's the PRHI-Toyota Production System principle that says the people doing the work know how to fix the work. They can be empowered to do it, and then the individuals that are engaged with them need to accept that work, test that it is in fact effective, and then implement it widely.

Within three months we have eliminated central-line-associated bloodstream infections in these two ICUs largely through the work of nurses, by engaging the patient at the bedside, and by creating counter-measures each time we found an infection to make sure it wouldn't happen again.

Now, our nurses have defined and implemented the best practice for dressing the lines and standardized the dressing kits we use. They document the current condition of the site every day, and they assist us in understanding alternative ways to do this.

FIVE ANSWERS

This is real-time observation. We began this process in July of this past year. We found four line infections that this team and I investigated in real time. We found that each of these line infections had a root cause. This femoral infection was due to leaving the line in place for a long time. You can, in real time, define what actually happened. This allows you to create countermeasures. And each time you do this, you can do it in a very quick period of time.

In the end, this allowed us to say: Here are the five things we want to do. We'll see if we can eliminate these infections. They are pretty simple.

No cost is associated with this first one. We think the subclavian is the best place to put the line. That's because it's associated with the lowest risk of infection.

Second, we believe that you should never rewire one of these lines. If you feel like you need to rewire a line, it's a call for help. It means you are struggling with how to get additional access. You should remove all femoral lines.

Third, on the door of any patient in our ICU with a femoral line there's a big sign that says, "Alert! Femoral line in place." placed at what hour on what day. So it's unambiguous to someone walking by when this line needs to come out. It's a signal that's unambiguous.

Fourth, we remove all lines that are present in patients when they are being transferred.

Fifth, every day on rounds we always ask the question "Do we need this line?"

PRHI and the Toyota Production System bring us here every day to do this work. They don't lead us to a conference room where six months later we analyze the data just to say we've looked at it. That's the difference between conventional performance improvement in a hospital and real-time performance improvement, which is the PRHI-TPS model.

198

By September 30th we had gone to zero infections. In fact, it's been 62 days since the last central line infection was recorded in the MCU or the CCU. It's doable. Zero is achievable. In doing so you honor the work of the people that are actually engaged in it.

CHECKLIST

There's a pilot-copilot approach where the pilot, the physician putting the line in, and the copilot, the nurse, are checking off a list of steps that they want to make sure they've carried out before they go forward.

All of this work can only be done at the bedside with the patient, as opposed to the conventional approach, which was to do these things outside of the room without the pilot-copilot approach that is so important. That's what makes sure that I double-check everything I'm doing with the eyes of another health professional who can guide me. No pilot goes down the runway without the copilot saying we're ready to go. That's the approach that PRHI has encouraged us to take in dealing with the placement of these central lines.

Richard Shannon, MD, Chairman, Department of Medicine,
Allegheny General Hospital, PRHI

One unexpected cause of central line infections was that the doctors and nurses had been trained at different schools—all of which taught different ways to insert and maintain central lines. The end product of this effort was that everyone agreed on a standardized way to insert and tend the lines. In the next chapter there will be more on removing barriers between doctors and hospitals

SOME THINGS TO REMEMBER FROM THIS CHAPTER

✓ A difficult shift for managers learning systems thinking is to understand and encourage the new role of front-line workers.

✓ Real-time problem solving by front-line people—people at the point of care trained in systems methods--saves lives and reduces suffering, errors and costs.

✓ Real-time problem solving is significantly more effective and humane than traditional management improvement committees studying the problems for months and then directing the front-line workers to implement the committee's improvements.

✓ This is because the front-line workers are closest to the problems and understand the work.

✓ They see the problems happening in real time.

✓ In the past, they may have been blamed for the problems, which they weren't trained to solve.

✓ Solving problems while caring for patients gives the front-line workers satisfaction and recognition and allows them to practice their healing vocations.

CHAPTER 17

REMOVING BARRIERS BETWEEN DOCTORS AND HOSPITALS

So far, we started to see some change but it's been very gradual change. It's very difficult to change physician practice patterns, but we're trying.
JoAnn V. Narduzzi, MD, Ph.D., VP, Academic Affairs,
Pittsburgh Mercy Health System, PRHI

A DELICATE SITUATION

In this chapter we look at a delicate situation in American health care, which is difficult to describe, much, less resolve. It is the problem of built-in opposition among the strongest elements of the healthcare system, specifically between the management that administers the hospital and the physicians and surgeons that perform their services there. PRHI and SSM Health Care have made some headway in resolving this dilemma, but it is still plagued with many areas of ambiguity. Barriers are reinforced by confusing payment systems.

According to systems theory, cross purposes among the people in the system make it less efficient and impair commitment to the system's avowed shared aim.

Among his Fourteen Points, Dr. Deming strongly emphasizes, when he counsels in Point 9, "Break down barriers between staff areas." In explaining this point, he writes,

> Often a company's departments or units are competing with each other or have goals that conflict. They do not work as a team so they can solve or foresee problems. Worse, one department's goals may cause trouble for another.

The major competing interests Deming found, when he consulted with American automakers, were labor unions and corporate management. They seemed to have different agendas, neither of which was to produce quality automobiles. The unions were interested in increasing worker salaries, benefits and, of course, job security. Management's goal was to maximize profits to keep shareholders happy and to maintain and improve the lifestyle of managers. It was an ongoing win/lose tussle between the two factions. As a result, the automobile buyer lost, both because of higher car price tags and poorer quality workmanship.

Deming felt their differences could be overcome and a win/win situation created for all concerned—labor, management, and customers—if both sides could commit themselves to making quality vehicles that satisfied and delighted customers. American automakers tried successfully for a while. But new leaders with different agendas, short-term goals and focus on quarterly profits reversed and effectively stalled the transformation.

A similar conflict of interest exists in most hospitals today between physicians and management. Systems thinking says, at least theoretically, that the conflict can be resolved, as Deming recommended, if both sides are committed to providing continually improving patient care. If caring for each patient in the best possible way becomes the primary task of both physicians and management, there should be no conflict. Or if a conflict arises, it should always be resolved in favor of the patient and what is best for the patient.

But not all doctors are systems thinkers and many do not want to put in the effort required to become a systems thinker. Nor are all doctors committed to the radical transformation of hospitals as described in this book, especially if it means they will have to make major changes in their attitudes, behavior, and mindset. And administrators are new at leading a hospital as a system. Most administrators don't know about systems thinking.

In this chapter, we get a feel for the slow but sure change of heart happening among physicians when they see the kinds of improvements in health care that are possible using systems thinking and quality methods.

However, unbalanced financial incentives, the traditional independence of physicians, and the sometimes fierce personal agendas on both sides keep the walls up between the two groups in hospitals that are not trying to improve systematically.

For example, an adversarial relationship can easily develop between physicians and the hospitals where they practice, because most doctors are not employed by those hospitals, but serve as independent contractors. They are not paid by the hospitals but by their patients or the health insurance companies that represent them.

If this were the airline industry, it would be as if airline pilots did not work for the airlines, but worked for themselves, were paid directly by their passengers, made their own schedules, and flew their planes however and wherever they wanted.

And some doctors do not view and treat the nursing staff as professionals.

At SSM and PRHI hospitals these barriers are breaking down. Nurses, physicians, and administrators, all trained in Toyota principles or CQI methods, are working side by side on teams to redesign procedures, eliminate medical errors, and reduce unnecessary deaths and waste. Change didn't happen overnight, and there was much resistance at first to this new system, just as there had been in the manufacturing industries.

But because everyone in the hospital system shared the same aim of perfect patient care, and the doctors could see that mistakes and suffering were increasing despite their best efforts, many of them began to realize they needed to take a different approach. But others resisted.

MEETING RESISTANCE

Clearly, at first there was resistance to this radical transformation. I think you're always going to have a medical staff that seems to be divided into thirds. The top third will go along with where you're going, they'll embrace it and they're eager to participate. The bottom third wants nothing to do with it. You can present all the data in the world and they're not going to change. That middle third are kind of the fence sitters, they can go either way.

Paula Friedman, Vice President, Systems Improvement,
SSM Health Care

Doctors are increasingly frustrated about a lot of different things, including the fact that they spend less and less time, in their view, interacting effectively with patients, really not doing the thing that they entered medical school and the profession for in the first place. The fact that all of the people who are involved in the healthcare process are frustrated about it sounds very familiar to people in manufacturing.

Cliff Shannon, President, SMC Business Council,
Pittsburgh, PA

RECEPTIVE HEALTHCARE WORKERS

However, continual improvement and systems awareness seems to be growing much more quickly, more deeply and more effectively in health care than they have in the American auto industry. Perhaps because physicians began to see that conditions were not getting better although they were working overtime and doing their best. Highly educated and motivated doctors and nurses are increasingly aware that something more than best efforts and hard work is needed to improve the quality of care and their working conditions. They had to learn and try something new. Systems thinking and continual improvement turned out to be the answer. But it came only after long years of frustration.

> Physicians, for example, do not believe that they will ever be able to get into an environment where they are not constantly hitting their heads against the wall to get work done efficiently and without error. They just do not believe it, because all through their training they had to work around obstacles thrown up by the processes of care that they were in the middle of.

Michael H. Culig, MD, Cardiothoracic Surgeon,
West Penn Hospital, PRHI

To make matters more difficult, hospitals and the doctors who work in them have confusing incentives concerning patient care.

MIXED INCENTIVES

> If you're an internist and you have a patient admitted with a myocardial infarction the hospital gets paid a fixed payment, whether the patient stays one day, two days, five days. But if

you're a physician, you get paid daily. So your incentive as a physician is to keep the patient longer. The hospital's incentive is to get the patient out. And it's just the beginning of the conflicts between the doctor's needs and the hospital's needs.

JoAnn V. Narduzzi, MD, Ph.D., VP of Academic Affairs,
Pittsburgh Mercy Health System, PRHI

What finally resulted at the two hospital systems was that, instead of focusing on the doctor's needs or the hospital's needs, they found a shared primary commitment to the patient's needs. In the above conflict, the patient's need became the measure of the length of a patient's hospital stay.

GETTING PHYSICIANS ONBOARD

So when we can show them data that these patients have better outcomes, they buy into it. Because physicians basically want to do what's right for the patient.

Paul Convery, MD, Chief Medical Officer
SSM Health Care/St. Louis

I felt as if much of what I did as a physician didn't matter. While I had good relationships with my patients, my ability to really affect their overall outcome was somewhat limited. So, like many physicians today, I felt powerless. I felt embroiled in issues surrounding medical legal matters such as the malpractice crisis. I was overwhelmed with the requirements of what payers in my institution wanted in terms of my documentation. I felt as if I was being further and further removed from the bedside. And I thought it was probably time for a change.

Richard Shannon, MD, Chairman, Department of Medicine,
Allegheny General Hospital, PRHI

Physicians will get on board if we can show that we can make life easier for them, and make the complex processes they perform easier to do.

Paul Convery, MD, Chief Medical Officer
SSM Health Care/St. Louis

205

At SSM, using the Baldrige Award criteria was another way of engaging physicians...and the rest of the staff. The next chapter explains how it helped more and more people to understand how they fit into the big picture.

SOME THINGS TO REMEMBER FROM THIS CHAPTER

✓ As reported earlier, the patient has gotten lost in the modern hospital; another unlikely victim of hospital complexity is the doctor.

✓ The doctor, like the patient, can be helped when the entire healthcare system agrees on an aim or vision of continual improvement of patient safety and care.

✓ Hospitals traditionally worked for the doctor and now that role must change.

✓ Doctors, unlike airline pilots, are not employees and they can do their work as they like.

✓ Doctors are so overwhelmed with new and conflicting information, new regulations and requirements, sicker patients, threats of lawsuits, etc., that many feel they have no time to investigate relatively simple improvements or reorganization of work.

✓ Hospitals must begin to collect and present data to doctors to convince them that systems thinking improvements will help them help their patients and themselves.

✓ Data also helps doctors recognize the seriousness of a problem before improvement starts—something they might not see from their own isolated practice without data.

CHAPTER 18

SELF-ASSESSMENT WITH
THE BALDRIGE CRITERIA

The thing that would improve American health care
is the use of the Baldrige criteria, and for the federal
government to recognize that not everyone has the
same access to health care as the people who are mak-
ing laws.

Sister Mary Jean Ryan, FSM, RN, President & CEO,
SSM Health Care

The Malcolm Baldrige National Quality program is a government and private sector partnership to help businesses, schools and hospitals learn to apply systems thinking and continual improvement to their organizations. They give national awards each year to organizations that practice their criteria.

The criteria, according to Harry S. Hertz, director of the program, show organizations how "to respond to current challenges and address all the complexities of delivering today's results while preparing effectively for the future."

Even if you don't apply for the award, the criteria provide any organization with a framework to help measure performance and plan in an uncertain environment. They help organizations—schools, hospitals and businesses—understand and apply management methods and theories. According to systems theory, the absence of a method or theory of how to organize work to achieve specific outcomes is one of the major reasons American hospitals are unable to reduce unnecessary deaths, errors, infections and waste even as advances in technology, pharmaceuticals and medical knowledge allow greater benefits.

"The Baldrige criteria offer an assessment tool and management approaches that help organizations improve communication, productivity, and effectiveness and achieve strategic goals," according to Hertz. Again, these same theories and methods are needed—and work—in schools and businesses as well as in hospitals. The American automobile industry's inability to apply such systems thinking, continual improvement and addressing customers' needs is the primary reason they have lost market share to the Japanese automakers.

AMERICANS TEACH THE JAPANESE

It was in Japan in the 1950s that these ideas were developed and tested by American statisticians W. Edwards Deming and Joseph Juran. Their assignment was to help the Japanese revive their crippled economy after World War II and help industries recover from a reputation for producing junk.

The Japanese culture is more cooperative and has a longer-term outlook than competitive, short-term, individualistic American and Western values. The Japanese took naturally to Deming and Juran's ideas of cooperative teams of people producing greater wholes, collecting data to describe problems and find root causes, and striving for unending improvement and customer satisfaction.

Meanwhile, America after World War II had the only intact economy, so desperate customers would gratefully accept products of whatever quality they could get from auto and appliance manufacturers. Poor quality products and services were not a good foundation or management mindset to be competitive in the late 20th or early 21st Century. Nor was it helpful to hospital administrators as American medicine exploded with new technology, organ transplants, sicker and older patients, huge hospitals and increased government and insurance regulations and paperwork.

This was what Sister Mary Jean Ryan faced at SSM Health Care in the 1980s when she knew that the SSM system of more than 20 hospitals across the Midwest had to improve, even though they were producing better results than the average American hospital. In 1989, she began to apply Dr. Deming's quality ideas of creating a culture of continual improvement and systems thinking. After a few years of practicing and teaching these ideas, she turned in 1995 to the Baldrige criteria to help her organization understand how it was doing and to better spread and share new learning and best practices through the hospital system.

THE QUALITY JOURNEY

Paula Friedman, SSM Vice President of Systems Improvement, explains this quality journey. "Journey" is how people and organizations pursuing and practicing these ideas often describe their continuing personal and workplace transformations.

> SSM started on a journey of continuous quality improvement in 1989. And it really was a long-term plan in order to improve how we do our work. We started to use the Baldrige criteria as a framework for process improvement in 1995, first as self-assessment and then throughout the organization in a more formal application. And it was done in an attempt to improve how we do our work in every aspect—from leadership to planning—to focus on the patients. Of our information systems, our staff and our processes, our day-to-day work, we asked: How can we do it better? How can we better understand our current performance and where we want to go? And how can we compare ourselves to best-in-class performers?
>
> The Malcolm Baldrige National Quality Award is premised on a framework for performance excellence. It is characterized by setting categories where an organization can look at its performance across the entire system so that it can achieve excellence, not just in singular areas, but across everything that it does.
>
> (The Baldrige categories are leadership, strategic planning, customer and market focus, measurement, analysis and knowledge management, human resource focus, process management and business results.)
>
> There is a series of questions within each of those categories that an organization asks itself to improve. And it was in the process of answering those hard questions that we really learned about what's important to us, how well we were communicating it across the organization and how well we were performing.
>
> Sister has been a proponent of continuous quality improvement in looking at the day-to-day improvements within the scope of a larger framework. So our evolution to Baldrige and the

use of that was a natural for her. Sister's ability to take day-to-day improvements within the context of a larger vision is what she's great at.

PARTNERSHIPS

Hospitals are intimately linked to the communities they serve and most believe they have a public responsibility to their communities. To operate a successful healthcare system, hospitals must assume the responsibility of collaboration with their communities.

> Sister is very much a proponent of collaboration. It becomes how we do our work. One of the questions in the Baldrige framework under public responsibility is: How can you effectively use partnerships and affiliations to help you in your organizational goals? Sister has always encouraged that. Every one of our hospitals participates in a healthy communities initiative with local social agencies and other partners, in trying to improve the health in the communities where they serve. So, for instance, our SSM rehab institute focuses on brain injury and spinal cord injuries. They will work with school partners in parishes in distributing helmets. But it's measuring not just how many helmets did we deliver or distribute throughout the year but what has been the effect on head injuries in the emergency rooms. And so it's the reduction of head injuries without a protective safety device, as opposed to an activity measurement of X number of new helmets per year.
>
> *Paula Friedman, Vice President, Systems Improvement,*
> *SSM Health Care*

THREE QUESTIONS

It has been said that the right question often suggests the answer people have been struggling to find. The secret is in finding the right question. One of the most powerful elements of the Baldrige system is that it asks just such right questions.

> If you look at the Baldrige model for instance, it has a whole section on focus on patients and other customers and it's how do you structure everything that you do to meet the needs of those that you serve. And when we talk with our managers

across the system, we ask them three questions. First, "Who do you serve and what do they want from you?" Second, "How do you know that you're providing what they need and how well you're performing?" Third, "What do you measure and monitor to know how you're doing and where you can do it better?" That's a fundamental issue that we can all benefit from. We all have people that we serve day in and day out, whether it's patients, other staff, physicians, the community, board members, whoever. But it's trying to understand their key customer requirements and how you can restructure the delivery of your work to make a difference.

Paula Friedman, Vice President, Systems Improvement,
SSM Health Care

BALDRIGE CRITERIA: DOCTORS AND NURSES CHEER THE CRITERIA

We have implemented CQI (Continuous Quality Improvement) at SSM Health Care since 1990. And CQI is the process and the tool that helps us make these improvements. But it wasn't until we began to use the Baldrige criteria that we were really able to focus CQI and link it to what we wanted to achieve and to really align it and drive it across the organization. CQI is a very valuable and useful tool. But you need something else to focus it, link it, and align it across the organization to get the kind of results you want to achieve.

Paul Convery, MD, Chief Medical Officer
SSM Health Care/St. Louis

BALDRIGE AND MONEY: THE ADMINISTRATORS LIKE IT TOO.

You can't win the Baldrige Award without showing great business results. As the first healthcare winner of the Baldrige, a lot of what that business model did was take our foundation of continuous improvement, give us a focus and a discipline to integrate these activities on what's most important for the patient and the family in a way that we were unable to do in the early part of our journey with CQI.

211

Thanks again to the Baldrige rigor and our efforts in continuous improvement we are also looking at our performance and employee satisfaction, patient satisfaction, position satisfaction and clinical outcomes.

William Schoenhard, Executive VP & COO,
SSM Health Care

RESISTANCE

We started going through the Baldrige, using its criteria as a framework for improvement, and people said, "Sister, we don't have time to do the self-assessments. We don't have time to write the applications. We don't have time to do this, we have other problems and fires to fight, and everything else." And Sister listened to that input but has always relied on her own internal compass to reply, "No. We are committed to this. I see enough improvement. It resonates with my personal values. I believe that this will help us become a better organization." And she has been the constant driver throughout the last 13 years at SSM Health Care.

William P. Thompson, Senior Vice President,
Strategic Development, SSM Health Care

THE SSM PASSPORT

Every SSM Health Care employee receives a Passport, a statement to fold and store under his or her identity nametag, which they wear at work. On it is printed the SSM mission statement and values as well as a list of the characteristics of exceptional health care service: "Through our exceptional health care services we reveal the healing presence of God." Below these, it contains empty lines for the employee to write in the shared goals of the hospital facility where they work and those of their department. More personally, there is also space to write in their own individual job goals and the measures the employee will take to realize them.

The Passport creates a connection moving upward from personal goals through departmental and facility goals to the goals of the total SSM Health Care organizational network. In this way, the Passport

Program ensures that all individual, departmental and facility plans are aligned with strategic goals and action plans at the system level.

SSM Health Care integrated their exceptional healthcare characteristics with the Baldrige criteria.

> Within the Baldrige framework, within the seven criteria categories, we have found that each is integrally linked to the other. Many people say that the hardest one is leadership. How do you identify, set and deploy what's important to you as an organization and make sure that everyone understands it? We have done that effectively through the development of passports and posters throughout the organization.
>
> *Paula Friedman, Vice President, Systems Improvement,*
> *SSM Health Care*

Posters displayed in each hospital show the linkage between department and facility goals. Managers identify department goals to support the institution's goals and assist employees in developing individual goals on their Passports to support department goals. This helps create and ensure the important system quality of alignment. Alignment means that every individual goal is aligned with their departmental goal, every departmental goal is aligned with its facility's goal, and every facility's goal is aligned with the overall organizational goal. In this way, everyone works in harmony, and the purpose of the whole is the purpose of every part.

> It's one thing to establish performance measures and goals at the system level, and it's another thing to ensure they are aligned at every facility, in every department, and with every employee – especially with 23,000 employees across four states. The thing is, you can measure and monitor performance 'til the cows come home. It's alignment that ultimately will drive your results.
>
> To ensure that this alignment occurs at all levels of the organization, each of our facilities develops goals that support our system goals. Then every department in every facility sets measurable and specific goals of their own, which support the facility goals. Departmental posters are on display. To support their departmental goals, all 23,000 employees in our system fill out

Passports, small cards that list their individual goals. These employee goals are a direct connection to our mission, because on their passports employees answer the question, "How do I provide exceptional health care services to our patients and other customers?"

This is alignment—a direct line of sight between every employee and the SSM mission. I can tell you from having seen it work that when every employee is focused on your mission every day, your organization will achieve results you never thought possible.

Sister Mary Jean Ryan, FSM, RN, President & CEO,
SSM Health Care

THE POWER OF ALIGNMENT

Let me give you an example of an individual's Passport goal and its potential to improve care. Here's the goal: "one hundred percent of the time, before leaving a patient's room, I will let the patient know I am going to leave, and I will ask if there's anything else I can do before I go." That's a great individual goal. Imagine if it's magnified thousands of times, so that 15,000 employees ask that same question of patients. The message that comes through loud and clear is: "We really care about you." And there's an added benefit. Let's say that when the nurse asks if there's anything else she can do, the patient says, "Now that you mention it, I'm uncomfortable, and I need help turning over." The nurse assists the patient before she leaves the room. As a result, the patient doesn't need to press the call light. So by asking a relatively simple question, the nurse reduces the number of call lights that come to the nursing desk. This simple act magnified thousands of times can make a profound difference not only in our patients' care, but in their perception of how well their needs are being met. Plus it helps our caregivers make better use of their valuable time.

Sister Mary Jean Ryan, FSM, RN, President & CEO,
SSM Health Care

EMPLOYEE SATISFACTION

Perfect patient care and better financial reports were important, but Sister Mary Jean believed that the foundation for these was employee satisfaction.

> Do I think that people have a right to meaning and joy in work? Well if I didn't, I wouldn't be here. But where I think this has to go is with every employee that we have. Every employee is entitled to meaningful work. We've gone a long way in being able to help with that by virtue of our mission statement and the way that we have cascaded it throughout the organization.
>
> Every single person in the organization has this little card, including me, called a passport. That passport provides me the opportunity to promise in specific and measurable ways what it is that I'm going to do every day to contribute to the mission. That's the meaningful part of it.
>
> The joy should come from people's ability to be able to change the work that they do, where they are, in order to make it better. And one of the questions that people are asked as part of Baldrige is, "Do you feel that you have the ability to change things that need to be changed?"
>
> *Sister Mary Jean Ryan, FSM, RN, President & CEO,*
> *SSM Health Care*

GETTING THE WORD OUT

The passports helped every employee know where they fit into continual improvement and fulfilling SSM vision.

> Our passport helps us draw a clear line of sight from our system's vision to our region's vision or our entity's strategic plan down to the person who's actually providing care or providing service in our institution. One of the good things of the discipline of working to earn the Baldrige Award has been clear line of sight that we have honed and fine-tuned and been able to draw. The passport is actually a tangible piece of evidence that says I'm linked to my hospital.

215

We describe our goals in three buckets: clinical excellence, financial performance and patients, staff and physician satisfaction. So my group that belongs in the exceptional clinical quality bucket says: A 50 percent reduction in the number of rejected blood specimens due to mislabeling in the emergency department and in-patient unit.

The second one is: one hundred percent of nursing units will have a shared accountability structure in place. The third one is: Increase physician satisfaction with nursing to 76 percent.

[The passport is] the link. How do I link to my department goals? My role is clearly a supporting role. I don't prevent phlebotomy errors by changing the way I draw blood because I don't draw blood. But what I do is support the team that works on rejected specimens and if the team says we need X, Y, or Z item to help support our work, I make sure that I represent the team to get that piece of equipment or whatever it is that they need.

Grace Sotomayor, RN, Chief Nurse & VP Patient Services,
SSM DePaul Health Center

MY PASSPORT GOALS

As the educator I fed my goals into our department goals for pain management and discharge instructions. My first goal is that 100 percent of the staff in my area would be educated on pain management and complete a pain management program by the end of 2003. And my second goal was developing diagnosis-specific patient education discharge packets by the end of the year.

The first one's done. And, everyone has been educated and completed their program. The diagnosis-specific education packets are nearing finish. They're being reviewed by other people for accuracy and to make sure that's the message we want to get out.

Grace Sotomayor, RN, Chief Nurse & VP Patient Services,
SSM DePaul Health Center

[Establishing and meeting such goals] is just part of what we do all the time. It's the way we do everything. It's incorporated. Everything we do, any change we make, anything we look at, immediately [we ask], "How do we know if this is going to work?" What can we do differently? If this isn't working, how should we change it? If it's doing well, can we do even better the next time? And if we do really well, can we share it with others or get some input from others?" It's just a part of what we do.

Diane Herbst, RN, Clinical Educator,
SSM DePaul Health Center

My personal goals are: I will look at 100 percent of my labs appropriately. I will label a hundred percent of my labs appropriately 100 percent of the time. That links to our department. There have been problems in the past with mislabeled specimens, specimens being in the wrong tube. My goal is to always look at everything that I do and make sure I do it right with my lab specimens. And my second personal goal is: 100 percent of my verbal orders will have verification or read-back 100 percent of the time. And I monitor that myself [to] make sure the doctor knows that I'm providing the care he expects.

Russ Schroeder, CTC Telemetry Division,
SSM DePaul Health Center

My first goal was to work with the staff to improve patient loyalty by visiting with the patient...and then to take it a step further, visiting some of the people that are admitted from here to the floor. Another goal was to meet with the physician staff regularly regarding their issues or to make sure that we were staying on top of the relationship between the physician and the nursing staff. My goal for improving employee satisfaction was to increase and improve my communication with them. Finding different creative ways to make sure that everybody felt like they were informed about all the things that they needed to know And then increase our shared accountability process. We've had several big projects that are shared accountability practice. We need to get the staff more involved in that sort of thing.

The shared accountability practice council is doing very well. Our patient loyalty scores are improved significantly. Communication between the physicians and the nursing staff has gotten better.

Kristine Mims, Clinical Director Emergency Department,
SSM St. Joseph's Health Center

The Baldrige criteria are an excellent, economical and accessible way to look at improving a social system such as a hospital. And remember, SSM was the first hospital or health care system to win the Baldrige Award

SOME THINGS TO REMEMBER FROM THIS CHAPTER

✓ The Baldrige criteria help an organization understand and apply management methods and theories.

✓ The absence or misunderstanding of management methods and theories is the major reason American hospitals are unable to reduce unnecessary deaths, suffering, errors, etc.

✓ The Baldrige criteria help organize and improve communication, productivity, and effectiveness and achieve strategic goals.

✓ If an organization applies for the Baldrige National Quality Award, the Baldrige examiners offer reinforcement, encouragement and practical advice.

✓ For SSM Health Care, applying for the Baldrige put their healing process into overdrive and spread it throughout their hospitals.

✓ Baldrige was a key factor in creating a new quality culture.

CHAPTER 19

OTHER HAPPY RESULTS

Continuous quality improvement happens every single day. By continuing to work with continuous quality improvement we can keep on improving our processes. It's sort of like healing the process. We are in the healing ministry to heal patients, but we ourselves also need that healing in our processes to see how we can make things better. CQI did that for us. It gave us a great sense of pride in doing something that we believed in the beginning was not possible and we achieved it.

Brenda Peterson, RN, Patient Access Director,
SSM St. Joseph's Health Center

Here are some of the happy results of the transformation processes being carried out in the two healthcare systems, SSM Health Care and the Pittsburgh Regional Healthcare Initiative:

◆ Their approach used simple and clear methods.

◆ The transformation did not require hiring experts to do the job but could be carried out by hospital staff.

◆ It was not necessary to hire new nurses and other health-care workers.

◆ It was not necessary to involve the government.

◆ The transformation did not cost additional money, and provides continuing substantial savings in money and time as well as reducing unnecessary suffering and death.

◆ The improvements keep happening.

◆ Staff know how to make improvements keep happening.

◆ Patients are happier.

◆ Doctors, nurses and other staff are enjoying their work more.

◆ Blame and fear are no longer part of the atmosphere.

◆ Every employee feels empowered to suggest changes and ways to implement them.

◆ Everyone in the system agrees that caring for patients is their primary purpose and is committed to that purpose.

We were like a lot of organizations in that we would try to fix problems by adding staff. That was always the first thing we came up with. We believed we could move this process along if we just added another nurse over here or another technician over there, or if we just added another room over here. What we learned when we spent that year developing our system was that our processes were flawed. Now when we want to solve a problem, the last thing we do is add people. The last thing we do is add resources. We look at our design and we improve our design.

Kevin Kast, President,
SSM St. Joseph's Health Center

We have been able to demonstrate to ourselves and others that patients on a pathway actually get better with fewer resources than patients that are being treated by physicians who believe they know best, who are relying on memory and training experience to do the right things for patients.

We are trying to recognize that most errors in the delivery of health care are not caused by the person but are caused by the system or the process in which he or she works. We recognized early that the 23,000 employees in our organization do not come to work thinking they're going to make a mistake or want to make a mistake. They want to do their absolute best job.

By focusing on the process and looking for ways to change that process and deliver better, more cost-effective care, the individual is freed. It takes the onus off individuals and allows them to apply their talents and skills and their creativity in a much different fashion.

William P. Thompson, Senior Vice President,
Strategic Development, SSM Health Care

So much in organizations is doing things because that's the way we've always done them. Now, we really assess why do we the things that we do. Everything that we do now is more intentional than ever before. We understand the questions of those we serve, what they want from us and how we know that. And we put that into place with defined measurements. So, it's not just delivering exceptional health care, but understanding how we define that and what that is.

Paula Friedman, Vice President, Systems Improvement,
SSM Health Care

People don't want to make mistakes, but sometimes processes in place can cause mistakes because of breakdowns from one department or another. So, what we do is focus on identifying the process we need to improve. We don't focus on the individual.

Maggie Fowler, Vice President of Patient Services
SSM St. Joseph's Health Center

When we started this 30/30 program in the emergency department, we knew we were only achieving the 30-minute time for patients at about the 60 percent mark. Now, we've been exceeding 90 percent for two years. So, if we added up the amount of time-saving for those 65,000 patients that we see on an annual basis, that might be a way to determine how much time we've saved—not only our time but the patients' time as well.

Maggie Fowler, Vice President of Patient Services
SSM St. Joseph's Health Center

We're not going to see healthcare delivery costs decrease overnight by a third, but I think we'll be able to reflect, a decade after we've started this activity in Pittsburgh, that in the community people are healthier than they would have been and more productive. And that the dollars that we're spending on health care in our community around Pittsburgh are being spent more efficiently, that people who previously didn't have access to care have more access to care or some access to care that they wouldn't have otherwise had.

Cliff Shannon, President, SMC Business Council,
Pittsburgh, PA

221

CQI has given us a mechanism to say to people when they walk into our doors, we value you as an important asset and contributor to our system. And we're going to provide to you the environment that allows you to flourish. Not only will you flourish but also it will help us achieve collectively the goals of this organization.

William P. Thompson, Senior Vice President,
Strategic Development, SSM Health Care

Our patient satisfaction that the call light was answered quickly was at about 92 percent last year, which was good. But we've got it to almost 97 percent so far this year, which means that a very large percentage of our patients feel their call lights are answered quickly. This, I think, gives them a sense of security that their needs are being attended to. And that's something that we share with all of the nurses in the staff meeting, and that always makes them very proud.

Diane Herbst, RN, Clinical Educator,
SSM DePaul Health Center

It's given me a newfound belief that, in fact, we can make a difference, we can change this. I believe that if we eliminated medical errors there would be no malpractice. I now believe, through PRHI, eliminating medical errors is entirely possible, but the work begins with us. The work begins at the patient's bedside. The work begins in collaboration with the people that provide the care. The work begins by listening to what they know about how to make things better, not the historical top-down approach.

Richard Shannon, MD, Chairman, Department of Medicine,
Allegheny General Hospital, PRHI

I just feel more energetic about my job. It has given me something to work towards. I feel that I have hands-on improvement in nursing. Also, I think it is good for nursing because it's cutting back on some of the drudgery of running around looking for what you need all the time. People become a nurse to take care of patients. They want to do the best job they can. The more time they get to spend educating patients and taking care of them, the happier they are with their job. And I think it's really going to help with retention.

Pam Seigh, RN, Clinical Supervisor,
Allegheny General Hospital, PRHI

It's a sense of accomplishment in having made a change that's been productive, that the rest of the staff find helpful as well. Sometimes we don't always adjust to change easily. But when it is a productive change and it's good for the patient and good for the staff, it goes a lot smoother and a lot easier. And I find that enjoyable.

Carl Glenn, RN, Surgery Staff Nurse
SSM DePaul Health Center

People don't like change, but at the end of the day, when they realize they're going to have more time to spend with the patient and less time looking for supplies and linens and answering the phone, I think it's going to make the work more enjoyable.

Connie Cibrone, President & CEO,
Allegheny General Hospital, PRHI

The CQI and our Baldrige efforts make this the most gratifying time of my life. From what I have been able to observe in the time that I've been in my position, things have not always been good. But what I have seen in terms of progress recently is something that, if I died tomorrow, I could die happy, knowing that we have a lot of work to do yet, but somebody will be here to carry it out.

Sister Mary Jean Ryan, FSM, RN, President & CEO,
SSM Health Care

I am convinced, had I not gotten engaged with PRHI, not only would I not be here, but I might not actually be doing what I'm doing today. Which is taking better care of my patients, feeling better about the work I do, engaging with my colleagues in a collaborative effort that is exclusively focused on what the patient needs. So, for me personally it's rejuvenated my career. It's kept me in Pittsburgh. It's kept me in this institution.

Richard Shannon, MD, Chairman, Department of Medicine, Allegheny General Hospital, PRHI

SOME THINGS TO REMEMBER FROM THIS CHAPTER

✓ The happiest result for these two healthcare systems was a radical shift from single-event thinking to systems thinking and seeing previously hidden connections, interactions and possibilities.

✓ Without systems thinking, improvements would have been mediocre and short-lived.

✓ Remember, a system is a whole, greater or less than the sum of its parts.

✓ Systems thinking allowed the hospitals to move toward being greater than the sum of their parts.

AND FURTHERMORE, SOME INTERIM RESULTS FROM INDIVIDUAL HOSPITALS:

- An estimated $1.7 million has been saved and fewer deaths caused as coronary bypass readmission declines 4.7 percent.

- There has been an 85 percent reduction in hospital acquired infections that are often fatal and cost $30,000-$90,000 each.

- There has been a 63 percent reduction in central line infections since 2001. Half of such infections are fatal and each cost $30,000+ to treat.

- Staph Infections were reduced from 26 per thousand patients to 8 per thousand.

- The significant mediation error rate was reduced from 0.16 per thousand dosages administered to 0.01 per thousand.

- Intensive care unit mortality was reduced from 5.5 percent to 3.3 percent.

- Acute diabetic complications were reduced from 13.5 percent to 5 percent.

- Administering aspirin in the emergency room for heart attacks increased from 40-50 percent to 95-98 percent.

SOME RESOURCES ON SYSTEMS THINKING AND IMPROVEMENT OF HEALTH CARE DELIVERY

CC-M PRODUCTIONS VIDEOS

(Go to www.managementwisdom.com)

The Deming Library (32 Volumes). Available in Spanish.

The Deming Revolution

How Everyone Wins: Finding Joy, Meaning and Profit in the Workplace

Better Management for a Changing World (Interviews with Dr. Russell Ackoff on systems and Dr. Gerald Suaréz on managing fear)

If Japan Can...Why Can't We?

CC-M PRODUCTIONS BOOKS

Dobyns, Lloyd and Clare Crawford-Mason, *Thinking About Quality: Progress, Wisdom, and the Deming Philosophy*, Times Business, Random House, 1994.

Dobyns, Lloyd and Clare Crawford-Mason, *Quality or Else: The Revolution in World Business*, Houghton Mifflin, 1991.

ARTICLES

Ackoff, Russell L. et al. al., "An Idealized Design of the U.S. Healthcare System," January 1994.

Berwick, Donald M., "As Good As It Should Get: Making Health Care Better in the New Millennium."

Godfrey, Blanton, Donald Berwick and Jane Roessner, "How Quality Management Really Works in Health Care."

Lambert, William J., "Health Care Quality: A Tale of Multiple Cultures."

Reinertsen, James L., MD, Michael D. Pugh and Maureen Bisognano, "Seven Leadership Leverage Points," May 2005.

Spear, Steven J., "Fixing Health Care from the Inside, Today," *Harvard Business Review*, September 1, 2005.

Spear, Steven J., Regina E. Herzlinger, Clayton M. Christensen, Richard Bohmer, and John Kenagy, "Curing U.S. Health Care, 3rd Edition (*Harvard Business Review On Point Collection*)," May 1, 2006.

Spear, Steven J., and H. Kent Bowen, "Decoding the DNA of the Toyota Production System" [Download: PDF].

Womack, James P. et al., "Going Lean in Health Care."

ADDITIONAL BOOKS

Ackoff, Russell L., *Ackoff's Best—His Classic Writings on Management*, John Wiley & Sons, 1999.

Ackoff, Russell L. and Sheldon Rovin, *Redesigning Society*, June 2003.

Ackoff, Russell L., *The Democratic Corporation—A Radical Prescription for Recreating Corporate America and Rediscovering Success*, Oxford University Press, 1994.

Deming, W. Edwards, *Out of the Crisis*, Massachusetts Institute of Technology, 1986.

Deming, W. Edwards, *The New Economics—For Industry, Government, Education*, Massachusetts Institute of Technology, 1993.

Institute of Medicine, *Crossing the Quality Chasm: a New Health System for the 21st Century*, July 2001.

Langley, G. J., K. M. Nolan, T. W. Nolan, C. L. Norman, L. P. Provost, *Improvement Guide: A Practical Approach to Enhancing Organizational Performance*, 1996.

Liker, Jeffrey, The Toyota Way: 14 Management Principles from the World's Greatest Manufacturer, McGraw-Hill, 2004.

Liker, Jeffrey and David Meier, *The Toyota Way Fieldbook*, 2006.

Ohno, Taiicho, *Toyota Production System: Beyond Large-Scale Production.*

Rovin, Sheldon, Neville Jeharajah, Mark W. Dundon, Sherry Bright, Donald H. Wilson, Jason Magidson, and Russell L. Ackoff, *An Idealized Design of the U.S. Healthcare System*, Interact Consortium, 1994.

Scholtes, Peter R., *The Leaders Handbook, A Guide to Inspiring Your People and Managing the Daily Workflow*, McGraw-Hill, 1998.

Scholtes, Peter R. et. al., The Team Handbook: How to Use Teams to Improve Quality, Joiner Associates Inc., 1988.

Studer, Quint, *Hardwiring Excellence: Purpose, Worthwhile Work, Making a Difference.*

Womack, James P. et al, *Lean Thinking: Banish Waste and Create Wealth in Your Corporation*, Revised.

THE BALDRIGE NATIONAL QUALITY AWARD:

www.quality.nist.gov

PITTSBURGH REGIONAL HEALTHCARE INITIATIVE:

www.prhi.org. An essential resource. See especially the "PRHI Executive Summary," a monthly newsletter.

ACKNOWLEDGEMENTS

This book and the accompanying documentary, *Good News: How Hospitals Heal Themselves* turned into a pro-bono effort by a former Peabody-award NBC television production team—most in their seventh decade. (One in his ninth.)

They wanted to raise a national discussion about America's grave patient safety problems and available straightforward, local solutions. Family and friends generously supported the team.

The project grew out of a 30-year collaboration among Lloyd Dobyns, former NBC News anchor, the late Reuven Frank, former NBC News President, and Clare Crawford-Mason, former NBC news producer. Together in the 1970s they had raised for the first time public discussions and awareness of a number of important issues, including spouse abuse, child sexual abuse and abortion as a political issue.

In 1980, they introduced the ideas of systems thinking and quality management to the West in *If Japan Can...Why Can't We?*

If Japan Can... featured Dr. W. Edwards Deming, who is credited by the Japanese with helping them recover from World War II. He taught Japanese export companies to "work smarter not harder" by introducing systems and quality theory and methods in the 1950s. This NBC White Paper was recently named the second-most influential documentary in the history of film and television by **The Washington Times.**

Twenty-five years ago, Robert Mason, who had been sent by the Smithsonian to Harvard Business School to bring modern management to the national museums, joined the NBC team. (He started the Smithsonian Associates.) Mason, married to producer Crawford-Mason, told the NBC team that Dr. Deming was saying something new and different than he had learned in business school. He then started CC-M PRODUCTIONS to explain quality and systems to American managers.

Over the years, the team produced many documentaries including the 32-volume *Deming Library* and *Quality...Or Else!* a three-hour PBS special in the 1990s showing how manufacturers in the U.S. and around the world were learning to work smarter. And there were books and seminars.

The hospital project, expected to take a year, began in 2002 when they decided to try to explain systems thinking to a general audience. (See the Foreword.)

Funds for documentaries, however, had dried up, but without fanfare. News documentaries, expensive to produce, had all but disappeared except for a few by network anchors who considered themselves journalists first and television personalities second.

The Baldrige Foundation, supporters of the Malcolm Baldrige National Quality Awards at the National Institute of Standards and Technology, gave initial start-up funds for the documentary. The Baldrige Awards have helped spread systems and quality ideas to American businesses, schools and hospitals. It is the only national effort to bring these important ideas to the country.

Howard McClintic of the CTC Foundation spent endless hours on the telephone and in person to generate support for the project. He was the youngster of the group, being well-below retirement age. His enthusiasm and diligence inspired the production team, which was greatly strengthened by Dr. Linda Doherty, formerly director of the U.S. Navy's Total Quality Leadership program and Dr. Louis Savary, who had written handbooks for *Quality...Or Else!* as well as over 100 books on other topics and, of course, this one.

Veteran network cameraman John Murphy, also the cameraman for *If Japan Can...*taped the interviews. Former **Life** and **People** photographer Dick Swanson, also a senior citizen, did most of the off-line editing along with Victor Crawford, Jr., who also designed this book and made countless changes as we practiced continual improvement. Karl Whichard was the on-line editor. Alan Foster uplinked the documentary to PBS stations.

We were blessed with advisors who reviewed our work: Dean Blanton Godfrey of the School of Textiles at North Carolina State University and Leona Schecter, our literary agent. And then there were the wonderful staffs at SSM Health Care and the Pittsburgh Regional Healthcare Initiative (PRHI).

And, of course, we want to thank W. Edwards Deming, Joseph Juran and Curt Reimann. Drs. Deming and Juran conceived, pioneered and developed these ideas of improving complex social systems over more than a half century. Dr. Reimann lead the effort to help American schools, businesses and hospitals practice them as he founded and oversaw the Malcolm Baldrige National Quality Award program.

A documentary and its non-fiction news book differ from other art forms. They follow the story as it develops. This story, healing hospitals in America and ultimately the rest of the world using systems principles, is just beginning. It is a change of culture and will require many more generous-hearted, curious, hard-working people as it continues.

We were fortunate to find an excellent first group of extraordinary talent to begin to explain it to a general audience.

This was the last documentary of the late Reuven Frank, legendary pioneer television newsman who invented the television news documentary in the 1940s. He brought wisdom and editorial genius as our consulting senior producer.

INDEX OF NAMES

AUTHORS:

LOUIS M. SAVARY holds a Ph.D. in mathematical statistics with applications in the behavioral sciences. For over thirty years as an author, lecturer, trainer, professor and workshop leader, his career has been dedicated to translating social and psychological scientific research into popular language. He is author, co-author, or editor of over 100 books. With Educational Systems for the Future, Inc., Baltimore, MD, as senior analyst and training developer, he wrote competency-based training materials for schools and industry. He created over 100 modules for General Motors, Dow Chemical and Federal Express, among others. With CC-M Productions, Inc., Washington, DC, he developed training materials applying systems thinking to organizational transformation following the approach of W. Edwards Deming: *Quality...Or Else! A Training Handbook* (CC-M, 1997). With Crawford-Mason he co-founded the Center for Directed Evolution, Inc., a group of scholars and business people investigating the next step in human intelligence and technologies for getting us there.

CLARE CRAWFORD-MASON is a journalist, television producer and author. Her 1980 NBC documentary, If Japan Can...*Why Can't We?* introduced W. Edwards Deming to the West and is credited with starting popular awareness of quality, productivity issues and the global marketplace. It was named one of the five most influential documentaries in television and motion picture history by The Washington Times and is used in industry and schools to explain these issues. She is the co-author with Lloyd Dobyns of two books on better management practices, *"Quality Or Else! The Revolution in World Business"* (Houghton Mifflin) and *"Thinking About Quality: Progress Wisdom and the Deming Philosophy"* (Times Books). She is the producer of the PBS series Quality...Or Else! used in companies and colleges to explain the problems of the global marketplace. She is the producer of the 32 volume Deming Video Library explaining Deming's theory of how to manage a complex purposeful social system in a changing world and the eight-volume Better Management for a Changing World video series, which explains systems theory and thinking, how to manage fear in the workplace and how to use the Enneagram in management and for a more fulfilling life. She lectures, consults and teaches workshops on various aspects of better management.

She was a founding editor and Washington Bureau Chief for 10 years of People Magazine. She reported from the White House from the Kennedy to the Reagan Administrations for television, newspaper and magazines. She was the first to report on network television and in a national magazine about spouse abuse (1975) child sexual abuse (1977) and abortion as a political issue (1979). She has won a Peabody award, two Emmys and was nominated twice for the Pulitzer Prize by The Washington Star and The Washington Daily News. She is co-founder of CC-M Productions and of ManagementWisdom.com.

The Nun and the Bureaucrat

EVERYBODY WINS

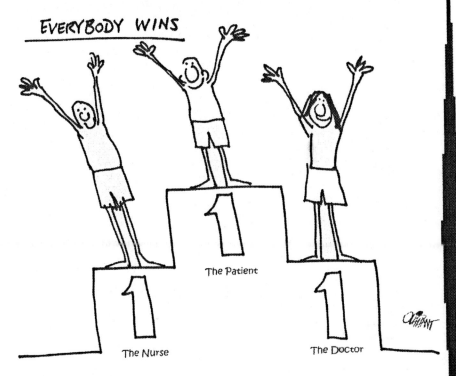

The Patient

The Nurse

The Doctor

HOW THEY FOUND AN UNLIKELY CURE FOR AMERICA'S SICK HOSPITALS

Companion to the documentary:
Good News...How Hospitals Heal Themselves
which is transforming health care

Louis M. Savary and Clare Crawford-Mason

THE NUN AND THE BUREAUCRAT

How They Found an Unlikely Cure for America's Sick Hospitals

Doctors, nurses and administrators explain how they did not believe they could reduce unnecessary deaths, suffering and mistakes by using systems thinking and Toyota production methods. To their surprise and delight, they did. They also dramatically reduced costs, increased their satisfaction in work, and required no outside funds or government help.

WHAT THE EXPERTS SAY:

If you think that hospital care cannot be significantly improved in quality and cost, you have another think coming. Read this book.

> Dr. Russell Ackoff, Ph.D., Professor Emeritus, The Wharton School. Author: Ackoff's Best; The Democratic Corporation; and Redesigning Society (with Sheldon Roven)

This book describes the kind of leadership that's essential for making our hospitals safe and patient friendly and at the same time cutting costs by driving out waste. And that is leadership that employs systems thinking to realize an inspiring vision. Read this book to learn how two leaders educated and transformed their hospitals. They show the way that others can and should follow.

> Michael Maccoby, M.D., anthropologist, psychoanalyst and consultant on leadership. Author, The Gamesman; Why Work?; and Narcissistic Leaders, Who Succeeds and Who Fails

If ever there was an idea whose time has come, this is the idea and this is the time.

> Cal Thomas, syndicated columnist (Denver Post, Baltimore Sun, etc.)

This book gives me hope that we can make similar improvements at many hospitals around the country

> Kenneth H. Cohn, MD, MBA, Cambridge Management Group. Author: Better Communication for Better Care: Mastering Physician-Administrator Collaboration

These authors have created an inviting introduction to health care as a system. In the midst of widespread recognition that we must improve our health care, they offer a starting point for creating the changes we need. Their attention to the insightful people making these changes happen allows us to learn from what's working. They have seen what is hard to see at first: health care as a system. Their writing is clear and inviting. In short, this is a welcome addition to the public conversation. Read it, share it and tell your elected officials about what you now understand needs to be encouraged to make health care better.

> Paul Batalden, M.D., Professor, Dartmouth Medical School

Louis M. Savary
&
Clare
Crawford-Mason

The Nun and the Bureaucrat

How They Found an Unlikely Cure for America's Sick Hospitals

CC-M
Productions,
Inc.

Printed in the United States
54667LVS00007B/115-510

9 780977 946105